POWER
of the TABLE

Roslyn Fisher, RNCP

ISBN: 978-0-9949461-0-2

DEDICATION

This book is dedicated to my family – my beautiful daughters Madison and Ryley, my husband, and love of my life, Chris and my step-sons Steven and Andrew.

CONTENTS

ACKNOWLEDGMENT

Since 2005, Highway to Health has provided me with the incredible opportunity to meet thousands of amazing individuals, each with their own compelling life story. This book captures many of the key themes I've covered with clients since then. It never ceases to amaze me how powerful the concepts are in REAL LIFE and it brings me joy to see the positive impact on so many. So for my clients, please accept my love and gratitude for who you are and for all your support.

Yours in health,

Roslyn

INTRODUCTION

The modern family is a tough crowd! There are so many expectations that we put on ourselves, from how to do, to what to do, and what not to do. With Facebook, Instagram, television, friends, and family, everyone has an opinion. In spite of all of these opinions and directions, everyone is trying their best to make it in this world while raising a family. And without a rulebook on how to raise our little creations, we need to roll with the punches and figure out what works. We learn from our mistakes, picking up the pieces and approaching situations differently, then getting back in the game. We wear all kinds of hats; we are moms/dads, spouses, friends, aunts/uncles, employees/bosses, cousins, brothers/sisters, neighbors, granddaughters/grandsons, grandmas/grandpas, nanas, and papas, and the list goes on. For most families, moms and dads are both working. They are also working longer hours than they used to, with expectations to work into the evening and on weekends as well. Add children into the mix, and the demands of raising the perfect family is way above and beyond a full-time job. We are grasping to find connection with people, a meaning for living, and a simpler way. Magazines and books hype the concept of simple—to just breathe and take time for yourself—but in all of this hustle and bustle, it can feel impossible to even simply stop to breathe. The family unit made up of several people all come with their own individual needs. Children have their own needs; they like certain foods, and they have demands, activities, and schedules they need to adhere to. Finding time for ourselves—what's that? How do we balance that into the mix? When does this craziness end? And now I am suggesting we sit down at the table each night as a family and connect? Ohh my gosh...STOP, I am not Martha Stewart, nor am I Super MOM. Can you just leave me alone already!

I see parent after parent come into my office who struggle to feed and connect with their children, and to find an easier way. They struggle with how their child should grow, are they growing too much, too big, or too slow? They are concerned with how much their children are eating each day, too. One child in the family eats too much, and the other child eats too little. Finding a meal they can put on the table that the whole family will enjoy is one of their biggest stressors. Some moms are even going as far as feeding their children first and then eating when their husband gets home later, to enjoy a quieter, more peaceful meal. Does this sound familiar? Families are, on average, cooking more than one meal each night; most are cooking upwards of three different meals and feeding their herd at various times throughout the evening. As a society, we are consuming more meals outside of the home, spending our disposable income on fast-food joints to simplify the frustration, confusion, and chaos of family meal time. It is no wonder families seem to have a schedule that is too tight to cook, spend time with each other, or find time for themselves. I had one family in my office recently tell me they had gift cards for a nice dinner place, and they wanted to treat their children. One of their daughters was very excited to go to the particular restaurant they had chosen, but their other daughter did not want to go at all. She actually put up a stink and started complaining there would be nothing on the menu she could eat. In fact, giving in to her demands sounds crazy when scrutinized, but we all do it in hopes we can have a more peaceful mealtime for once. Or how about this: a child running around the dinner table, jumping on the couch, or having a conversation from the other room while everyone else is trying to enjoy their meal. And think of the mom or dad struggling to prepare these meals. How does it feel for them when nobody likes what is being served or children act out, complain, or flat out refuse to eat? The use of negotiations, bribes, rewards, and punishments for eating or not eating is a valued practice in most families that leads to disconnected families and an introduction into emotional eating following these children for a lifetime. If you suffer from emotional eating—rewarding yourself for a good day or sabotaging yourself for a tough day—you can relate to choosing to teach your children a different way, developing a positive relationship with food.

As a society, we are struggling with raising the perfect child; the child who looks perfect on the outside. They are the right size, wear the right clothes, and they do the right things so they can fit into societal norms and expectations. Through this pressure, we put more focus on weight and growth, saying things such as my child is too skinny or overweight, they eat too much, or they eat too little. And through this process, parents are now finding themselves limiting food or bribing their children to eat. This emotional eating rollercoaster that families are on needs to STOP, and it needs to STOP NOW. We need to put an end to the cycles and patterns of weight loss programs, scales, overeating, under eating, emotional eating, and binge eating. Let's take one family at a time to a place where we can simply allow our bodies to take the lead, eating when our body needs fuel and stopping when it does not. As parents, we become so worried our children will look different to their peers or not fit in, and we may anticipate problems with bullying. But if we really sit back, break it all down, and think about it, if we all let our children just be children and allowed them to grow and discover at their own pace, we would all develop positive children who love and adore themselves for who they are.

Just a couple of weeks ago at my daughter's soccer game, I could see the parents in front of us were arranging a playdate with their daughters after the game. You could tell they didn't know each other well. I could see one mom arranging the car seat and some bags for the playdate. They were chit chatting about pick up times and who would drive home. It was all loosey-goosey. They seemed pretty laid back about everything, and all was good. Just before leaving with the children, one mom asked, "Does Isabella have any food allergies?" (This is the new norm these days.) The dad piped in eagerly and said, "No, but she is a really small eater." He continued to add urgently, "Isabella is really picky. REALLY REALLY PICKY." He continued to clarify his case so it could be heard loud and clear. He seemed very concerned they needed to know this. And it seemed odd that his concern was just then coming to the forefront. With the loosey-goosey playdate plans, this was such a huge deal. As I got thinking about it, what was he even telling these parents? What does picky eating have to do with food allergies, or better yet, having fun at a playdate? The reason why the word picky is being used so frequently is to protect parents. Parents are forced to understand their child's pickiness for fear their child won't eat, won't grow, or for fear their children will become upset and cause a big embarrassing and frustrating scene if something they do not like is served to them. What if Isabella starved at this new friend's house for the couple of hours she was there because she didn't like what was being served? Would that stunt her growth? Would she suffer? These may have been some the dad's concerns.

Or another concern could be what if they served her something she didn't like, and she started to act out or even cry? That would be embarrassing, and the dad may feel bad or hurt for her. At least by telling this family his daughter is picky, they will accept it. Why will they accept it? Because this new UNIVERSAL word is recognized and given a stamp of approval so everyone who encounters a picky eater knows what to do and what to expect.

This is absolutely insane. We have hit a decade of the pickiest of picky eating monsters and we are creating it, accepting it, and living with it. This emotional eating rollercoaster is allowing picky eaters to take over, to take control, and throw mindful eating out the window. We are catering to our children's palates, while our lives are becoming overwhelmingly stressful and as a family we are becoming more disconnected. Families no longer use the hub of the family table to reconnect and grow together. In fact, families fear dinner meals together and go to all costs to avoid them. I have clients who grab a sub after work and park in a parking lot by their home so they can eat in peace and quiet before going home to face their children. I have men who purposely or subconsciously come home late from work to avoid the uncomfortable dinner table, grabbing something on the way or reheating their meal when they get home so they can eat alone...and in peace. Families are simply passing each other in the hallway of their homes coming and going, and when they do finally sit down at the table, they are disconnected, getting up and down, eating over the sink, running off to activities, and utilizing their devices or watching television to get through their family meal together. Let me tell you right now, there is a much better way. There is a super simple way to get back to the table and stop the emotional eating cycle. None of us want our children in weight loss programs or developing anorexia or bulimia. We need to stop the pattern of using food and the numbers on a scale to control our emotional well-being. Developing the Family Table will free you to develop positive connections with your children and the food you are eating, which, in turn, allows you to enjoy your food and your family. As you read through my book, you will be amazed to discover that your task as a mother or father is simple—really simple—when it comes to feeding your children. And when this simple technique is downloaded and installed into your family unit, everything else in your lives becomes easier, too. Can you imagine never having to worry about dinner, about what you will make and what will happen at the table? Can you imagine never worrying about eating dinner at a friend's house, with the in-laws, or at a restaurant? Can you imagine your child never having to worry about their weight or using food as an emotional balm for lack of happiness or security?

The simple technique I will discuss trickles down to every aspect of your family. It changes how children feel about food, using it to nourish their bodies without the use of rewards and bribes or because they deserve it.

This technique carries down to how children feel about their bodies, positively affecting their self-worth and self-esteem. And all of this begins to happen when a Family Table is established. So simply read, and listen to what I am telling you, and follow each and every step consistently along the way. Throw the excuses and the doubt whether this will work out the window, and just trust me as we take on this journey together.

1 THE TABLE

What happened to those old traditional family meals where we used to all sit together at the table? We all knew how dad's work day had gone; we connected over what was new and what we had to look forward to. I remember when we were young, my mom would hold off on us eating dinner until my dad came home from work, so we could all sit together as a family. It was a regrouping time, a connection time, and the one chance we had every day to sit and talk to each other. Dinner was simply the excuse to get us to that connection. I know in my own family, the table is the only time we get to be present together in one room, facing each other, conversing, and laughing. Some of the funniest things come up at the dinner table, and I have never laughed so hard as during those times. How open our children are with us and the questions they ask are unbelievable to me, and usually something I would never have imagined bringing up to my own parents. We have created a safe haven, a comfortable space where nobody is judged, bribed, rewarded, or punished. When a safe haven is established, children open up, and this allows their bodies to get full nourishment from the foods they are eating. This safe haven is called the Power of the Table. Without the dinner table, it is almost impossible to get this same daily connection with your family.

When was the last time you ate a meal together as a family? Why have we created this lack of value for the dinner table? Is it because we have our children booked into so many activities, running them here there and everywhere over the dinner hour? Is it because moms and dads are working long hours to make ends meet? Or is it because we have now accepted the universal word "picky"? Is social media framing the way we should look, the way our children should look, and how our children should grow? Are moms and dads stressed and feeling overweight, tired, and themselves undernourished as they tackle caring for their modern family? Are we texting too much and using social media and television to entertain our families instead of having conversations that form connections? Are moms and dads suffering through the agony of preparing dinners the family won't like, or are they preparing many meals according to the likes and dislikes of their children? It's exhausting just writing about all of the things our families tackle in a day. We are disconnected, lost, and running more than ever before. Do some of these scenarios ring true in your family? The reality of the NEW modern family needs to change. We cannot keep living like this. We are losing our family unit and the connections our children need so badly in order to develop and grow properly.

The other day, I caught myself commenting on my daughter's Instagram picture. She had a photo of herself and me, and it read, "I have a great mom, and I love her more and more each day." It was so adorable to read; a statement over social media about ME as a mom. So I couldn't pass up the opportunity to respond on her page and wrote, "You are the most amazing girl! I love you to the moon and back! XOXOXOX."

She later opened my eyes when she said, "Mommy, why don't you just tell me that instead of typing it there for me to read?" She was absolutely right. We use social media to reach out to our friends, and sometimes we use it to reach out to our children, too. I want to be part of her world, but I also need to remember that as I am typing these things, she is often right there in the room, and the words I say in a live connection are more sincere than a typed message on Instagram or a text.

The dinner table is about forming connections with our babies, toddlers, children, teenagers, and spouses. When we are connecting and completely safe and content, we are able to digest the food we are eating more efficiently, absorb it, and nourish our bodies. Healthy bodies come from eating in a complete balance of peace and happiness. This whole philosophy I am presenting has nothing to do with what type of food, how much food, or how little food is being eaten, but everything to do with how the food is being presented and how parents are feeding their children.

Think about it. Would you feel at peace if your spouse constantly told you to take three more bites before you could leave the table or criticized you for eating too little or too much? Or what if he spoon-fed you with helicopter noises to get a few more bites into your mouth? Or said you needed to lose weight so you shouldn't have any more to eat? Or simply turned the television on to distract you so you would eat without complaint. How would you feel if your spouse punished you, threatened you, or told you there were no more helpings of rice until you finished two more bites of your broccoli? Or if your spouse actually took his fork and started dividing your food so you could get a visual of how much you needed to eat before you could say you were finished? Seriously, how would that make you feel? Would it make you feel small, unsafe, and insecure? What if your spouse finished their meal and they got up from the table while you were still eating? Would that make you feel lonely, disconnected, undervalued and unhappy? Maybe this happens in your family or happened to you as a child, and you already know how this feels. What if your spouse jumped on the couch, sat on your lap, crawled underneath the table, ate off your plate, wanted to be spoon fed, or actually got up and went into another room while you were still eating your meal? Would this make you feel disengaged, unheard, and misunderstood? Do you think your children feel this way too?

The other day, my daughter and I were eating breakfast together, and during the week, this is a time we aren't typically able to sit as a family and eat. Instead, this is a time everyone eats around the breakfast nook at their own pace so they can make it out the door on time for school. With the rituals of morning routine, my children are able to get up and get ready for school when they are finished. This one particular morning, I decided to eat with my daughter. And when I noticed she was finished, I told her she could go ahead and get ready for school. She looked at me with her big brown eyes, confused, and said, "No, mommy, I can't get up yet because you are not done. I am going to wait for you to finish." What my daughter was really saying was that she didn't want me to eat alone. Taken aback by her response, but at the same time, comforted and secure in her desire to keep me happy and safe while I finished my breakfast, I simply said, "OK, and thank you." I could safely say, in that moment, my job on this planet was DONE. If we learn anything from the Power of the Table, it is about connecting with each other, being in the moment, and feeling valued. A sense of unity is created, regardless of how much, how little, or what food is being served.

Are you using food for survival, to hide behind your emotions, as a control mechanism to reward or punish yourself. Or are you using food to simply bring people together to connect? Now don't get me wrong, food has valuable nutrients, and without it, we would not survive. But when we are connecting, we are nourishing our bodies with the food we are eating in the most healthful, flowing, and gloriously freeing way. The process of taming the monsters we have created around the table can be simplified with ease. What I am proposing is that it isn't about what is being served to our families; we can let that go out the window right now. It is about the type of eating environment we create in which to nourish our family's bodies. We are simply using food as a foundation to get us to the table. Through this philosophy, we use food, our number one necessity for survival, as a platform to bring us to the table, to sit at the table, and to stay together at the table for a period of time. The table is the one place where families can be close, see each other, and hear each other while providing their bodies with the necessities of life. You can serve take-out pizza for dinner and have the most amazing connection with your family. The idea of cooking extravagant meals every night to produce these lifelong connections and get your children to eat is no longer a positive method that leads to positive lifelong results.

As we go through life with our children, we need to pinch ourselves at how fast time flies. Our little babies grow into children, pre-teens, teens, and then adults.

And if we spend too much time scattering around, we will miss connecting, building a foundation, and growing together with our children while finding the true purpose for our own lives. As you follow me on this journey, you will see how the Power of the Table is all you need to raise positive young children and form strong family relationships. That's it! Together, we will first calm the rush of your life so you can begin to also calm the rush of your child's life and get your family connected again.

I will take you down the road to a happier, healthier, and more fulfilling family life while nourishing your own individual soul and body. Travel with me as I share with you my family who together, have developed a simple life of fewer distractions, more experiences, and a stronger connection all starting at the hub of the table.

2 HOW IT ALL STARTED

I began my journey at the young age of ten years old when I began babysitting. During the summer months while I was at University I looked after multiples as young as two weeks old. I would also come home on weekends and breaks throughout the year and care for children while their parents vacationed. Doing this, I was able to gain a lot of experience working with children as well as an understanding about how they behaved and developed. I had been exposed to hundreds of them. I loved children and knew exactly how to care for them. I remember pulling up to the local private school once in a borrowed Land Rover to drop off the girls I was looking after. One of the teachers came up to me and said, "I don't know what you have done with Sarah this week, but she is a different little girl. Whatever you are doing is working, keep doing it" I still remember that as such a huge accomplishment; I thought, "Yeah!" Be in control and be consistent was the name of the game.

I graduated with a degree in Applied Human Nutrition from the University of Guelph Ontario and went straight into opening up my own play group-based child care business called Happy Children in Healthy Families. There, I looked after children for a couple of years, cooking for them and planning programs in a calm, supportive environment. Shortly after I had my first beautiful baby girl, I completed my designation as a Registered Nutritional Consulting Practitioner and began my own practice, helping individual clients nourish themselves.

I dreamed my whole life of having a family. I wanted lots and lots of children. I got married at a young age and couldn't wait to be a mom. But soon, that picture perfect vision was shattered. My marriage wasn't what I thought it could or would be, and being a mom wasn't what I had envisioned either. My dream of a family had been different from the reality I was living. By the time my second beautiful baby girl came along, our family simply coexisted.

We never fought, because coexisting meant we knew what to do to keep living and surviving. That is truly what it felt like—survival. We went to work and juggled the bills and daycare smoothly while I switched my away-from-home job to a work-from-home job in order to keep the survival train going. Weekends were much the same. I made my work life coexist with the children's schedule, and life just carried on. We had very few of the same friends and had very few people over to our home. Our home was a secret, where we survived and lived as smoothly as we knew how. We did our own thing, with little fulfillment or happiness. We never fought or showed signs of distress in our marriage that would indicate something was wrong.

We were a picture perfect modern day family, and because of that, I should have been happy—at least that was what I was taught. I was always told marriage isn't perfect; it was the message I received right up to my wedding day, so I just accepted the unhappiness part as one of the imperfect flaws of our marriage and used what I saw of other peoples' relationships to justify that mine wasn't so bad. We loaded our days with lots of distractions: perfect family photos and few experiences.

Even when we went on vacation, we packed it with stuff; meeting new people was a number one priority the moment we got to our vacation destination. We took lots of excursions, partied, and danced the night away to mask how we really felt. The beautiful places we went to should have been enough, but I was still scattered, disconnected, and unfulfilled. I felt exhausted all of the time. I knew I wasn't the best mom to my girls, but I was managing the best I could, and I was overwhelmed at the thought of this being my life forever. I lived with a pit in my stomach, a feeling that something wasn't right. I knew I needed more, and I knew there was more out there for me.

So I explored myself for quite some time, to fully search for what I needed inside that awful pit in my stomach. I wanted that deep connection for myself and that deep connection for my children, too. I knew once I discovered my own happiness, meaning, and purpose in this world, I would be a much better mother to my children, helping them to fulfill a beautiful life, too.

I had gotten married at twenty-three years old, and when my marriage dissolved after ten years, I felt sad, lonely, and scared. The magical life I wanted was out there for me. I just needed to believe in it.

I just got remarried, in July of 2014, to the man of my dreams. My rock, the most caring man in the whole world. He is patient, sincere, and follows a passion for my dream. He too wants to fulfill his happiness and build positive, supportive, and nurturing relationships with his children. When we first spoke about getting married, it felt complicated. But as we thought about a simple approach to share our love for each other with less distraction, we came up with a marriage ceremony in our backyard, to ultimately follow our dream of a simplified life. So as we put this together in our backyard scenario, we came up with the bare bones we needed to form this marriage. An officiant, two witnesses, two rings, and of course, ourselves. Our wedding was perfect in every way; in the backyard of the home we built with complete focus on our marriage and our life together. I am on cloud nine as we continue to bridge our family together; our blended family is taking shape, with two terrifically caring boys, fourteen and twelve, and two sweet and loving girls, six and eleven. We are becoming a family unit who connect, have experiences, and laugh in the simplest of ways.

Now don't get me wrong, this bridging of our family has been a challenge. It is tough work to bring families together. Even between my two girls and me, we find our energies clash at times and it is tough to get along. Other times, we go through several months of staying in a groove that flows and feels easy. I love the word easy. With each bump in the road, I embrace it as an opportunity to grow and transition together into a new normal that keeps our beliefs and simple strategies at the forefront. As a family, we get through the storm to see the sunset every time. We have sought counseling together to understand our different personalities, and we continue to do so when needed. We connect with warm distraction-free conversations and experiences. We do this by making the dinner table a priority in our family. On weekends, we make all three meals - breakfast, lunch, and dinner – each its own event. The more often we can get to the table together, the better it is for our connection as a family. Meal time togetherness is so powerful. Throughout this book, I'll share with you my experiences and will help you and your family understand the Power of your Dinner Table, too.

Each chapter will follow a step-by-step approach to get your family back to the table. Once we get your family to the table, you will discover that other things in your life begin to come together easily and smoothly, too. Remember it isn't about simply eating together; it is a whole system. The table can be the safest hub for your family to reconnect, build positive relationships with each other and to discover healthy foods.

3 FAMILY

As I search for the words to describe our family, I come up with this: We trust each other, and we love each other equally and consistently. We are a flowing unit who connect for hours daily and thrive off of each other's support. We continue to honor our feelings and share with each other what those are. Although our home is made of brick, it is a cushion of safety for all of us. We feel safe and secure in our family home.

So to begin this journey, we need to consider what a family is to you. Does your family coexist? Do you come and they go? Does your family connect together? Take this opportunity to think about, or even write about, what your family is now and possibly what you want your family to be.

I asked a number of people, both men and women, this question: "What is family?" Approximately half the people didn't respond to my request and still have not responded. A quarter of the people had to take time and get back to me, and the other quarter responded within a minute of asking. I actually had someone e-mail me a week later, mentioning that they hadn't forgotten about my question and would get back to me. Another person said, "It is too deep for me."

It is a deep question, and if you have never taken a moment to reflect on your family or what you want as a family, it can feel uncomfortable. The variance in responses I received brought me to this conclusion: If you don't know what family is to you, then how can you raise the family you want? Typically, we are formulating our family based on what others, our inner critic (the nagging voice in our head), or our extended families think or expect from us. We use distraction and busyness to keep us from reflecting or feeling within our family unit. I have seen families pretending they are the family they want when out in public, but behind closed doors, it is an entirely different story.

Here is what some people told me a family is to them:

"Family is the people who surround and support you, building you up in good times, and bringing you back up when you are down."

"Family to me is a group of people who love and support you through the good times and the bad. They take joy in your success and happiness, and stick by you through tough times. They love you no matter what, just as you are."

Another person said family is, "Love, laughter, kindness, thoughtfulness, funny."

"A family is a group of people who love, support, and trust each other; who are there to celebrate the good times and to support each other through difficult times. Family also holds you accountable for your actions, speaking to you with love when you are going down the wrong path or participating in bad behavior."

"Family is a group of people you can draw from or share life with. Loyalty, honesty, protection, comfort. The one place I can be myself; no guard, no agenda."

"Family are people who will always stand behind you, support you in the toughest times, and love you unconditionally."

The other day, my husband and I were able to sneak

away and get lunch together. We went to an upscale restaurant in our neighborhood (a chance to eat without kids and chat about our stuff). We were seated beside a family with children. Mom and dad had a six-month-old daughter and a three-year-old son; Nona and Nonno were there as well. The baby was being held by mom and the three-year-old was in a high chair beside Nona. I had to ask my husband to give me a second just to get this scenario down for my book as I could see it unraveling. Thank goodness he is so supportive and understanding. I took my notebook out, grabbed a glass of wine from the waitress, and spent three minutes max (I knew it was our lunch together) taking notes on this family.

So here it goes, the three-year-old was the only one at the table who had his food. I guess the family ordered the little boy's food first so he could eat before everyone else. Nona (I am pretty sure that was what they were calling her; I am a terrible eavesdropper) was feeding the three-year-old to give mom and dad a break, I am guessing. She was hovering over his highchair, spoon feeding the boy, who was flat out refusing to eat. Dad was on and off his phone, drinking a beer, while from across the table, mom (again, holding the baby) and Nona were paying close attention to the number of bites and amount of food the three-year-old boy was having. "You like this, Aidan," they kept saying in unison. "Aidan, you need to eat," was another line coming from mom. Suddenly, the little boy got hold of daddy's phone and that was when the fun began. "You can't be on the phone while you are eating, Aidan," they said, taking the phone away. Meanwhile, Nonno, who was seated at the table, was on a phone call that continued for the entire meal, and I never did see him eating; and daddy was on his phone texting and watching the television screen across from him, piping in every now and again to encourage and possibly convince Aidan to eat. Mom continued to hold her baby girl, who was as cute as a button, and who wasn't old enough to eat adult food.

Soon, pizza for the adults came to the table, and Aidan wanted to try their food. The answer was "NO, Aidan, you need to finish your food first." Aidan had a mound of food to finish in front of him before he could have pizza, so there was no hope in hell he would get to have a slice. Good luck with that, I thought to myself. I kept telling my husband they needed my business card!

With that, the mom switched seats with Nona and took charge of feeding the little boy. Before the switch of seats, I heard her say, "Fine, Aidan, that's it. No more restaurants."

"Was she serious?" I thought. Aidan can't go to another restaurant. Mom sat down beside Aidan and tackled the exhausting chore of feeding her son. She began by asking him what napkin he would like on his lap and where his water was. I think she was trying to butter him up to eat. That took a solid five minutes to get set up. Meanwhile, Dad piped in, "You need to eat Aidan; come on Aidan, let's eat." You could tell the dad sensed the mom was going to blow a gasket, and he wanted to keep things calm, reminding Aidan in a subtle way, "Eat, or you know what happens to your mom."

Mom dove in with the spoon, loaded with some concoction, and Aidan refused to take a bite. After more tries, threats, bribes, and negotiations, mom had had it. She pushed Aidan's chair away angrily from the table in frustration (close to us now), and said, "Fine, if you are not going to eat, you can sit over there."

In fact, he had been the best behaved three-year-old I have ever seen in a restaurant. He just sat there in his exiled area and looked around for about twenty minutes…confused, disconnected, and sad. He then got pushed back to the table, where they tried again to get him to eat, but by then, he was crying. He didn't want to eat, and mom was MAD. Dad felt terrible for his son, saying, "It's OK, buddy."

But mom dragged Aidan, screaming and crying, out of the restaurant and to the car.

Take this family scenario, a family who loves their little boy so much that they just want him to eat and grow. This poor mom has become so consumed with getting her son to eat that the dynamic of the entire family table has changed. It has changed from connection, conversation, safety, and fun to a place of control, distraction, threats, bribes, anger, and tears. Dad has resorted to getting on his phone to escape from the reality of the family dynamic and speaks few words for the entire meal, while Nonno is disconnected and proceeds to talk on his phone for the whole lunch hour. Maybe he was just there to pay for the meal. The table has become an uncomfortable place for this family, and for many families, this is the same scenario every single time they sit down to eat. Remember how I mentioned most families want to look like everything is all good on the outside, but behind closed doors things change? The above scenario may be more intense at home, when nobody else is watching! And possibly even more intense when mom is alone, without support or watchful eyes. The chore of feeding their little boy has gotten the best of this family, leaving blood boiling day after day.

Now that I think about it, my own family also sometimes falls into this trap. We do look better on the outside than on the inside. Our children have access to their phones when home (except at the table or during family activities), but when we are out in public, the phones and other devices do not leave the house. Why is that, I ask myself. Am I also trying to portray a different family outside of my home than the one on the inside? Why do I strive to want to connect with my family more outside of the home and away from phones? I bring up this example because we all have something we can work on. So as we strive to achieve the family we want, there are many roadblocks that can get in our way; friends, devices, extended family, televisions, differences in personalities, work, school life balance, extracurricular activities, and our own personal development, to name just a few. Because of juggling all these balls in the air, we look to one place that is a constant. A place that delivers a truly meaningful connection each and every day. That place is the powerful table. We find the power of the table when we simplify our lives, eliminate distractions, and allow ourselves to be present.

In the chapters to follow, we will explore three topics that will help us get back to the table and see how very important this hub truly is.

4 SIMPLIFY

As I started down this path to a more fulfilled family life, with fewer distractions, more experiences, and less stress, I found myself simplifying things in my life. For me, this meant spending less frivolous money and time in the kitchen, taking the drama out of my life, running around a lot less, and having fewer meaningless things to move from one space to another space in my home, car, and office.

Fewer things

I shed light on this recently as our family began the process of less clutter and less stuff! I found when my house was a mess, I would become very distracted, at times angry and frazzled. I would spend my time moving items from one space to another space and continuing this process almost daily. Often, I remember saying, "I just cleaned this house up, and it is already a mess!" So I began taking it upon myself to conquer each room and closet, filling bag after bag of things we never knew we had. And as I dropped bag after bag off at the depot for donation, I began to feel lighter, less stressed, and less overwhelmed. When I entered into my home, I was looking at a cleaner, more organized space and I knew where everything was. Even my pantry was organized...I had food in there I never knew I had. As my space felt clean, my life and how I operated in it felt cleaner and, therefore clearer, too. It was a crazy phenomenon. I remember one time as I was dropping items off at the donation depot, another couple was there doing the same thing. With each bag the lady took out of her trunk, I could see how much lighter she felt. Her face, her body, her expression, and her energy were all lighter. I said, "Doesn't it feel great?"

She replied, "Ohh, yeah!" with a cheery voice and a great big smile. So I asked myself, if it feels so great, then why do we continue buying more things, cluttering our homes and our minds? Why are birthdays and X-mas about stuff and not about the experience and the connection? How many times have you thought and thought about what gift to buy someone and come up with the response, "They already have everything"?

By focusing on having fewer things, you make room

for more meaningful connections in your life. I caught light of this when my house was a mess. I would become distracted, angry, and upset. My energy would change by just walking through the front door of my home. When my house is clean and organized, with less stuff, I feel light, energized, and in control.

I was amazed by this feeling, so I did some research to see how real this feeling actually was, and this is what I found:

"Professional organizers who are called to cluttered homes and offices say their clients use the same words over and over to describe their reaction to the same mess. Their energy is drained, they can't find things, and it begins to interfere with crucial parts of their life, such as getting to work on time or navigating staircases." [1]

Can you believe that if you cleaned up and de-cluttered your space, you would be able to navigate crucial parts of your life better and your energy would increase? This same site suggests that "clutter is bad for your physical health. It can be a fire hazard and accumulate dust, mold, and animal dander. Clutter also changes the energy in your home." [2]

As I pondered over the stuff I did not want coming back into my home, I began to consider the idea that having less brings a feeling of lightness, less stress, and an increase in energy to me and to my home. When energy is heightened, it allows for a higher connection. In the process of simplifying our lives, I had the children go through this de-cluttering experience as well. I simply plopped down a box in the middle of their rooms, and had them start to form piles; piles of things they wanted to keep and things they wanted to donate. They needed to get the pile down to a size that would fit into their box and to only hold onto the items they absolutely loved. It was a fun process and something they were able to do on their own. This gave them confidence and control over their own belongings and what was valuable to them. When their space was clean they also looked lighter and less stressed, and they wanted to hang out in their new clean space more often. Their energy changed and the energy of their space changed, altering their enthusiasm for cleanliness. With just this simple exercise of fitting what you want into a box, I often find the children de-cluttering their space on their own. And what an amazing feeling that is to experience—children who want clean spaces, yeah!

We do this every few months. Because our needs change and our attachment to things change too. For artwork, I have gotten the kids a scrapbook they can glue their favorite pieces into. Every couple of months, we go through the art box to narrow down some more of what they want to keep or get rid of.

While doing this de-cluttering process, I was even able to determine that my home office was being used as a storage room. When I went in and tackled the space, I was able to move my entire office to a small wall unit in our home. It was crazy to me to see the amount of useless crap I was throwing into my office. Now that my office/storage room is cleaned out, my husband and I have a whole new sitting room in that we use to chill out in. We have gained more space, just like that!

And when asking a few people around me what "stuff" represents to them, this is what they said:

"Material items are a substitute for love. It is easier for some people to buy their kids stuff than it is to show them love with a hug or sit down and show care, compassion, sympathy, and empathy."

"Causes distraction, creates sources of conflict, takes away from family."

"Stuff/toys do not formulate a family—all that stuff means nothing—most important is love."

This Christmas I began to feel the anxiety of bringing more stuff, in the form of presents, into our home. So where there is anxiety, comes a solution. So I posed this question to my daughters to see if they would like to go away and have an experience with me instead of receiving material gifts that contributed to more meaningless stuff and more things to clutter our home. I said, "If we do plan a girls' trip, I would like the trip to replace any items you may get for Christmas and your birthday this year." I gave them the option to choose what they would prefer. It took them all of ten seconds before they both begged for the trip and the experience of being together and sharing a memory in lieu of more stuff. Their quick decision shocked me. But I was also happy with their response.

We booked a low-roller trip to Cuba, where we simply just HUNG OUT together. The only item we purchased on our entire trip was a deck of cards. We enjoyed playing cards before dinner; the game Old Maid was so much fun, and as I write this, I can still see my daughters' energy as they would hide their expression and keep their secret of the Old Maid being in their hand. We simply swam, read books, ate great food, danced, and napped, with no expectations but to experience each other. At one point, I caught myself telling the girls to just simply breathe the fresh air as I took a deep breath in and exhaled. Upon returning home, my oldest understood why I did that. The sense of freedom, relaxation, and simplicity took over on our trip. The other day while getting ready for bed, I caught my six-year-old looking at her pictures from our trip. She must've taken close to a half hour looking at every single detail and reliving the memories. Since coming home, my oldest, who is eleven, keeps asking if we can have that experience again. I love that my children are learning to simplify their lives in these easy but profound ways—taking away things and formulating experiences.

So how do you start to de-clutter your home? Well, it is very simple! Start small and tackle one drawer at a time or one closet at time. With each item you let go that no longer brings you joy, begin to feel your energy shift within your home. You will begin to feel lighter and more clear. Get help from your family members to do this. Give them some responsibility to clean their own spaces and keep them organized, and offer them tools to keep up with this process. When school bags, coats, etc. come home, give your children an organized space to put these items that is out of the way. It doesn't have to happen all at once, but once you tackle one drawer, you begin to tackle another, and the feeling becomes contagious. Try it and see your energy shift and the pieces of your life fall back into place.

Spending Less Money

As we continue down the road to simplifying our lives, the thought of spending money frivolously comes into play. My husband and I plan our weekends with our children with a focus on spending less. This dawned on me one weekend a couple of years ago, when I discovered how much money we were actually spending on meals out and entertainment on the weekends and how little I felt about the experiences we were having. It just became matter of fact, this is what we do. Instead, we did a mind shift to spend less money while achieving stronger, more meaningful, connections. Each weekend, we all try to attend one of the children's soccer and hockey games together. It is so nice to have all five of us cheer on seven-year-old Ryley as she saves a goal. Or the excitement of seeing twelve-year-old Andy power skate to the end of the rink and score a goal as he raises his stick and gives us a hand pump in excitement. It isn't just attending the game that brings us together, but it is the support we all have for each other on the way to the game and on the way home. We play street hockey, have family soccer games, play board games, walk to the lake, go skating, swimming, bike riding, and hang out in the back yard making wood oven pizzas and roasting marshmallows on the open fire. We make sure that each of our experiences requires less money or is free, for the most part, so we can focus on each other and our experience together. "I love free", I often say to my husband. On Christmas Eve this past year, we pulled out the game Clue. A brand new game we had not played yet. We had so much fun with this game. We played three rounds that afternoon, and then when we came back from skating that same day, the boys asked if we could play the game a couple more times. We got to spend three more hours that day, including meal times and skating, connecting, laughing, and being together without the big spend.

That day, we also decided to arrange a neighborhood hockey tournament. The e-mail went out the day of, and each of our neighbors showed up with sticks and nets for a fun-filled hockey tournament. It was so nice to see that one of our neighbors even took it upon himself to wear a referee jersey and be the ref for the game. Man we needed that. The game was one of the best memories we have made, and further connected us to our neighborhood. So often, families are going to great lengths to spend money at amusement parks or walking through malls on weekends. We got away from this and instead adapted the scenario of what can we do that is free or cheap. When we focus on FREE it becomes less about the distraction and more about our experiences and connection together.

As we focused on spending less money, we ditched going out for dinner and fast food was gone. Instead, we save our money, and purchase the best high-quality food to have meaningful delicious meals together as a family (and it is still far cheaper than going out). A week of groceries for us is one meal out. When we purchase food, we purchase only the food that is on sale. We scope the grocery store for the fruit and vegetable sales and the meat discounts before planning our meals. When chicken breast is on sale, for example, I will purchase several packages and freeze them. I never, ever buy regular priced strawberries! My husband especially loves to cook. Just this past weekend, my husband took a low-roller dinner of peanut butter and jam sandwiches, veggies, and drinks in a picnic basket to the boys' hockey game. Some kids ate in the car, some at the game, and some after the game. We weren't able to eat together at the table, but at least we were able to provide a fast healthy option that felt good and stuck to our formula of simple and free.

Now when we do have the opportunity to go out for dinner, we go all out. We go to the restaurant with the best vibe and yummy nutritious food so we can experience our connection together over a longer length of time. Going out for dinner is so rare, so it has become really special for the kids. They truly appreciate the experience, and respond with lots and lots of thank-yous!

When you like being together, it doesn't matter what you are doing. So start little by little to form these connections at parks, in your back yard, or in your own home or car. Keep it really simple and take in the formula of FREE!

Less Back and Forth

I explored how to make my time make more sense. How to become more organized. What was I doing that consumed my day? When was I booking the kids after-school activities? What was I doing in my business that distracted me? How was I spending my time with friends? Figure out what is holding you back. I had a look at all of these things this past year and made some changes.

I used to cook meals for clients. I love cooking, but the meals began to consume my day, and I became overwhelmed and consumed with cooking and meeting the demands of my business. So cooking meals had to be put to rest to open up more opportunities for me. I remember telling my husband, "I was so busy cooking today, and I could not get to the stuff I wanted to get to." Bingo, there was my answer!

I make time for me. With everything going on, you can begin to feel scattered at times, so unplugging, going for a walk, and doing what your body needs will help to stop the back and forth and chaotic to-do lists and chatter in your head.

I make a list. A list works well; before heading out the door, I make a list so I can tackle errands in order to get the most done in the least amount of time.

It's your schedule, not theirs. We allow the kids to choose one extracurricular activity a season. With four kids, that is enough. Because we skate, ski, bike ride, and the list goes on, as a family, it is important for me to be able to leave time for my sanity, meal times, and connection. I hear so often from parents that they live in their car. They are driving here, there, and everywhere, feeding kids at different times, etc. I invite you to take a look at your schedule and take small steps to make a schedule that works for you.

What will simplify your back and forth? What takes up the most time in your day? What is stopping you or getting in your way of doing what you truly would like to do? Take some time to make a list and cross off a few things that no longer serve you.

Less Time Cooking & Planning Meals

Here are some tips that have worked for me to spend less time cooking and planning meals and more time doing things that really matter.

Groceries: I plan my dinner meals for the week each Sunday. I plan three consecutive meals (after looking at the inventory in my fridge and freezer) and make a small grocery list. I choose three meals because often the plan can alter if you plan for more than that, and food can go to waste.

I cook less. I have learned that I do not need to cook gourmet fare every night for dinner. Eggs, pancakes, cold plates (cheese, crackers, hummus, veggies, beets and boiled eggs) all suffice and add the same value when connecting the family.

I cook in bulk. When I do cook, I triple my meal. We eat one for dinner (and sometimes as leftovers for lunch) and I store two meals in the freezer. For example, when I make homemade hamburgers, I make twenty-four burgers and freeze the extras. The same with meatballs, chili, and whole chickens (I cook two whole chickens and freeze the remainder).

I make rollover meals: I have learned to roll my meals into something else. Nobody loves leftovers, so why not take the leftover cooked hamburgers and make hamburger soup. Or why not take the leftover whole chicken and make a chicken casserole, chicken noodle soup, chicken curry, or chicken salad.

Before getting everyone to come to the table for meal time, I make sure I have everything we need at the table before sitting down. This saves the back and forth from kitchen to table and the disruption, too.

Finding your Life's Purpose

When you find your life's purpose, you begin to formulate why you are here on this planet and focus on that instead of dealing with the nit picky drama each day can bring. You begin to focus on the bigger picture and what really matters in your life. What is your purpose for living? The dryer breaks or the hot water doesn't work, but really, does that matter??

The other day, I woke up to a very cold home. Immediately, I convinced myself that because it was really cold outside, our heat must not be working as well. But soon, the heat really dropped. Instead of going into my normal "panic mode", I went on with my scheduled appointments and meetings and bundled up. I wasn't going to lose sleep over it. I didn't even feel the need to tell anyone about it, or make it part of my day. I picked up a fireplace for the basement at the local hardware store in between meetings, to warm up our home in the interim. My hopes was my husband could put it together before we went out for date night (we do date night once a month, so this was a big deal). Because time was limited when he got home from work, we decided to leave the assembly of the fireplace, enjoy our date night together, and deal with the heat issue when we got home. It flowed with my pattern for that day. Continue on and the rest will follow. Well did that ever turn out to be true. We had a blast at the movies (haven't been without kids in ages), and when we got back home, we walked into the most amazing energy. A warm house! I kid you not. The heat somehow magically popped back on—seriously! It was pumping! It was the most joyful experience I might have ever felt. To feel that basic necessity of heat! That was it. That was all we needed in that moment ("if we could only have heat"). Seriously, it was that simple.

And the best part was the excitement we felt; true excitement (I am not sure what other word to use for this) was what we felt. We kissed and hugged each other; turned on music and danced. We were joyful and truly blessed. It was surreal, and we were able to continue our date night with a nice romantic dinner.

When I woke up the next day, the heat didn't work again, but I was able to continue to feel and remember that high from the night before. The blessed feeling. Getting the heat fixed that day, whatever it meant, for us was not a big issue at all!

So when you formulate that statement of your life's purpose, really think about what makes you tick. Is it your job that gives you purpose? Is it your home or your family. Is it your happiness? What gives you your purpose? We tend to think about this at funerals or when we have a sick family member, or our child runs a high fever. You begin to understand what really matters. But sometimes that can be lost and forgotten in the day to day rush and chaos. So take this time to slow down, see, and truly feel and believe in what your purpose is.

Take a pen and paper and make a statement that sums up what you want to get out of life; what do you want for your children? What do you want them to learn from you? You will find it isn't about the big house or the fancy car or the amount of friends you have; it is much simpler than that. Once you develop this statement, your life will feel really simple. A load will come off your shoulders. You will say, "Really, that's it? Why am I always running after something more, something better? If this is my life's purpose, then I have everything I need right here."

You have everything you need within you. The drama, gossip, and possibly the judgment you feel from others, will go by the wayside. When you determine your life's purpose and really read it out loud to yourself several times, you begin to grow and connect with the people in your life who support your true self. It is a really cool phenomenon. Since formulating my life's purpose and reading it to myself several times, I now have so much more time on my hands to do what matters to me, my headspace feels cleaner and clearer, and my life has taken on a much simpler approach.

Take the challenge to simplify your life and begin to see things change around you. You may notice when you simplify things you begin to feel different. Your energy may shift. You may notice that you have more time to dive into other things that matter to you, or you actually have time to relax and take a breath—imagine that! Start with yourself first and take the load off, literally! Start with YOU and then work on helping your children. Master one technique at a time, and give yourself the time to sit with it before you move onto the next simple technique. I call this your sweet spot. Find your sweet spot, the inner light within you that shines and you will begin to live a more simplified life. Your family will live one too.

5 DISTRACTION

We can all relate to the hustle and bustle of a school morning and all that goes along with it. One Monday morning, I was getting myself ready for work and my children ready for school when my youngest daughter decided it was the perfect time to distract me. She wrapped her arms around my legs from behind as I was trying to locate something in the fridge immediately stopping me in my tracks and cementing me to where I was standing. It was one of those squeezes that take the breath right out of you.

In the rush of getting ready for school, that distraction may cause some moms and dads to get upset, because it disrupts routine. It literally caught me off balance. I call this a "routine interrupt." I remember it was at a time when I was really busy with work, leaving the house after the children were off to school, and rushing to pull myself together to give daily presentations to professionals. I forced myself in that distracted moment to put focus on what was actually happening, and I paused and took a deep breath in. Was she really trying to be a nuisance, or was she needing me close at that moment? Was she helping me to slow down, breathe, and stop for just a few minutes or even a few seconds? Her little hands squeezed around my body so I could not move, absolutely pinning me from moving any further. She was preventing the rushed exit to work and school.

In that moment, I took a deep breath and asked her, "Do you need a hug?" She quickly let go of me with a huge grin, came running around in front of me without a response, and wrapped her little arms around my neck as I lowered down to her height. I responded with, "I really needed a hug too." And as I thought about it, how else was she going to get my attention as I was running here, there, and everywhere around the house other than to almost throw me to the ground? She squeezed me and told me how good I smelled. She then said, "Stay like this, mommy."

Man oh man, she was even saying all the right things—the exact things I needed to hear to calm me down from the busyness I had created. I stayed there as she rocked me gently back and forth before she finally released me. Wow, did that ever feel good, I thought. It completely melted my heart to have someone give me permission to just stop, let go of distraction, and embrace. My life purpose flashed through my mind like a movie. One of my life purposes is to build healthy connections with my children, with less distraction. I took time that day to reflect back on what had happened. I looked back on my distracted busy life, and realized how many times my children would hug my legs while I was making dinner or on the phone or finishing an e-mail and I was just too busy and too distracted to notice. I sometimes felt frustrated they needed me during those busy times in my life. Kids always seem to act out and get your attention when you just got on the phone or have something important to get done. But is it only at those times they are acting out, or are those the times we typically notice it? I can confidently tell you one thing, kids don't just choose the busiest times to make the biggest fuss.

And it was upon this reflection that I realized I needed to change how distracted I was. I needed to let some things go to make room for what really mattered to me. I made a vow to myself that day that I would always make a consistent effort to listen and immediately let go of distraction for my children. To bend down to their level and look them in the eye when they spoke to me. And if I needed to send an e-mail or talk on the phone, I would be sure they knew I needed some time for me and that I would be all ears and eyes when my task was completed. It always amazes me how things hit us. It was a simple squeeze from my daughter that morning that opened my mind to a new way of living.

Distraction comes in all sorts of ways, from scattered and busy thoughts, daydreaming or from overworking ourselves and hyperextending our time with friends and family. It can also happen when we procrastinate and then become too busy and scattered to support our family when they need us. These are all escape mechanisms. If my daughter wrapped her arms around my legs when I was scattered, too busy, and distracted with tons and tons of stuff, thoughts, and chaos going on inside me, her arm wrap would have gone unnoticed. I would have asked her to move out of my way and get ready for school. I might have even had to raise my voice to really get to her, because sometimes kids can be persistent when we continue to ignore their cues.

It sounds terrible, but for you to find the truth of your distracted ways, I need to be truthful with you as well. How many times do you answer a question for your children and you have no idea what they even asked? Or do you hear your child calling your name a few times, failing to hear them until they have called you for the tenth time? The rock solid truth is parents are feeding their children, and themselves for that matter, in this same distracted and busy way, too—too distracted and too busy to eat, to notice, and to care.

I have categorized distraction into six main categories to narrow down what is going on inside all of us. I explain these in more detail below.

1. Busyness Distraction

I once lived a very busy life; one with little reward and a never-ending to-do list. I always felt like I was behind the eight ball, trying to get caught up on the things I had to get done in order to get to the things I wanted to do. At the end of the day, there were never enough hours. Weeks, months, and years would go by and my busyness continued. I struggled because the busyness that once fulfilled me, didn't anymore. It left me feeling discouraged and defeated each and every day. I wondered why that was. Why could I never keep up? How could I possibly keep living that way? My body felt like I was living in fast forward, but my brain always felt like it was moving in slow motion, and that to-do list never seemed to end. There was always something that needed to get done. I always wondered when the chaos would stop, until it dawned on me that I had control over this.

By putting myself in a constantly busy state, I was simply forming a fake distraction for myself. My busyness could be anything, and often it wasn't productive. I would take on more duties at my children's school, say yes to everything, pack my days with lunch dates and coffee dates that brought me back to busy on the other end. I was often hitting the grocery store once a day, sometimes twice, and hitting the bank once a day too...why?? And I just never stopped doing laundry until recently. This story is an interesting demonstration of how things do happen for a reason. My dryer broke down, so I was bringing my wet laundry to my parents' home once a week to dry. Initially, I couldn't understand why I didn't call the dryer fix-it man right away. With my schedule, I needed to do laundry every day, and if I missed a day, the stress and busyness would build. But instead, I took on the challenge of taking the wet laundry to my parents' home and thought I would leave the dryer repair for another day. It actually didn't get to me at all like it would have in the past, and I knew there must be a reason for my carting laundry back and forth. By bringing all of my wet loads of laundry to my parents' home, I killed two birds with one stone. I had more opportunity, while my laundry was in the machines, to build connections with my parents and my children, and all of my laundry was washed, dried, folded, and put away in one day. Prior to this, laundry in my home was on an assembly line twenty-four hours a day. Laundry would clutter my home, with some dirty, some clean, some needing folding, some still wet in the washing machine, and some folded in baskets on bedroom floors. Laundry was all part of my busyness. What a relief it was to find a new way. And now that my dryer is fixed, my new laundry routine is liberating, it doesn't consume me and it only takes four loads instead of the feeling of endless piles of laundry, and I am done for the entire week! Plus, the energy in my house feels cleaner and clearer because of this!

My business was also a source of busyness distractions. I was doing things that made me busy, but saw no end result. I recently went from a large 3,000 square foot studio to an office space I work out of one evening a week, and I work from home now too. WOW, what an unbelievable change, and the end result for my business is so much more rewarding because I am able to have the time now to focus on the areas of my business that fulfill my life's purpose. And when you fulfill your life's purpose, you experience great rewards, pleasure, and satisfaction from how you live your life. You ultimately feel aligned, at peace, and balanced. I believed that by being busy, I was made to feel more valuable and more respected, and in turn should have been happier. If I was busy, then I was giving and doing something, being someone. Busy people can appear to have a sense of stronger purpose. They can seem like strong individuals who can take on a lot. I walked right into this trap because I was hiding my happiness and what my true life's purpose was. For some, it can be because we are afraid or we simply just do not know. The light that shines within us can be scary. We are afraid we may be exposed and vulnerable to the world; we may shine too much, turn people away, or cause people to feel uncomfortable. Being busy didn't make me happy, but it somehow built an imaginary foundation and belief that someday it would make me happy.

How many times when talking to a friend do you hear them say, "I am just so busy." And when you sit and think about it, the only one who is making their life busy is THEMSELVES. Nobody else. But the busy excuse and the too tired excuse are distractions that people have grown to accept as normal.

We are over-scheduling our children and ourselves. Busy schedules load up our days where we are running here, there, and everywhere, leading us to distraction and leaving us with fewer moments to stop, breathe, reflect, and think.

When I stopped to nail down what was making me busy, it was a number of things that weren't satisfying me. They didn't align at all with my life's purpose, and some of the tasks were monotonous and made no sense when I really looked at them closely. As I examined every task I had going on in my life, from my business, home life, even down to cleaning my house and the time I spent volunteering, with my family and out with friends, I began to discover that a lot of what I was doing was filling time, giving me little satisfaction, and taking me away from what really mattered to me; taking me away from the things I wanted to do, the things that aligned with my core values and my beliefs. I soon realized, as I began to make changes and do the things I wanted to do, I didn't feel busy anymore. I felt fulfilled, nourished, free and happy.

2. Mental Distraction

Mental distraction is when the brain is overwhelmed. This could be due to all-consuming thoughts and ideas, brain fog (which can be from food allergies/sensitivities or due to alcohol or medications), daydreaming, stress, and exhaustion.

Stress and Exhaustion

Often, when we have high stress, our brains become overwhelmed and thoughts come in and out of our minds constantly. We may feel more energetic, move faster, or feel jittery and scattered. We might feel overwhelmed, that there is just too much going on inside of us, and have trouble sleeping or wake up for two to three hours in the middle of the night, wide awake because our mind will not turn off. We may stay awake at night, distracted with thoughts, ideas, and to-do lists that persist in our head. After nights like this, we feel exhausted and scattered the next morning, and the vicious cycle continues. Our body pumps up the adrenaline when we are tired from little sleep, and even more so when we exercise and are tired, to keep us up and energized throughout the day and into the night. We again wake up exhausted, scattered, and overwhelmed, and the cycle continues to repeat itself. To decrease mental distraction, I suggest finding a bedtime routine that will give you eight solid hours of sleep a night. If you can't find this time, then lost sleep needs to be made up on the weekends by sleeping or napping. Your body needs to shut down and your mind needs to calm. Adrenaline stored in the bloodstream is a very powerful and harmful substance and continuous and repeated surges of this hormone can cause a lot of health problems, from the insomnia we're talking about here to more harmful effects such as nervousness, lowered immune response, or an increase in insulin release leading to diabetes and obesity in the midsection. As well, a child with high adrenaline will have a more extreme reaction to every noise, will fidget, talk excessively, and have abnormal sleep patterns. In adults, adrenaline can speed up the signs of aging and these adults can look burned out or appear older than they are.

If you have this difficulty, some things to try to calm yourself before bed is take a bath, read a book, or listen to guided meditations. Avoid caffeine and alcohol in the evening to facilitate a more peaceful sleep. I would suggest that all screens get turned off an hour before bedtime. Getting enough sleep will calm your mind the next day, make you more mentally alert, decrease headaches, and also decrease your consumption of sweets, carbohydrates, pop, and caffeine that all act as stimulants to release adrenaline into the bloodstream. Simply by increasing sleep and paying attention to your sleep routine, you will stop the vicious cycle and increase your productivity.

Overwhelmed Thoughts

Remember that never-ending to-do list I was speaking about? When you get the right amount of sleep, decrease busyness, and decrease stimulants such as pop, diet drinks, coffee, tea, and energy drinks, you are able to calm the thoughts in your head. Thoughts can also be calmed by talking some sense into yourself. Often we play out scenarios in our head and assume the role of other peoples' thoughts. Instead, just worry about you and do not take on the thoughts of others, because you will never know what is going on in their head, anyway. Another great way to control overwhelming thoughts is through journaling; I talk about this often. So just go out and get a special little book, or a big one for that matter, where you can get your thoughts out of your head and down on paper. I use this technique a lot. I find this technique really clears my mind and gives me some perspective and clarity on what is really going on for me. Other solutions are Reiki, chakra balancing, yoga, meditation, and being outside in nature. All of those things will help to control the overwhelming thoughts that can go on in your head.

Daydreaming

Do you catch yourself daydreaming? Wishing you were

doing something else and imagining things differently in your life? This type of fantasy can be very distracting when it plays like a broken record in your head. To make sense of these distracting thoughts, use a journal to get these thoughts out of your head and down on paper, form a vision board (a vision board is a collage of pictures, phrases, words, or items that represent you and your goals) and clear your mind of this distraction and start making sense of your dreams!

Brain Fog

This is categorized as symptoms of forgetfulness, confusion, and lack of focus or mental clarity. Often an individual feels they are in a haze, depressed, or have a hangover type feeling. Brain fog can happen when the body has trouble eliminating toxins. A change in diet and consistently getting eight hours of sleep a night will change brain fog immediately. Again, if eight hours of sleep a night is a challenge during the week, sleeping in on weekends and napping is a must to make up lost time. A lack of sleep is a whole other ball game when it comes to a healthy body and mind. A lot of diseases would be eliminated if people just started listening to their bodies and got a good night's sleep. So just sleep!

Mental distraction does not have to be avoided entirely. It can certainly calm you down from what's ahead; a big presentation or a dance recital. Meditation, yoga, and massage can be used to calm the brain and take the load off your mind. Children like to play make believe, where they are daydreaming and escaping reality for a little while. We have acquired these resources to protect ourselves. But be aware of these mental distractions, and again, consider using a journal to write down what is consuming your thoughts. Getting them out of your head and down on paper is really helpful in making sense of what is consuming you. I also enjoy walking in nature to can get ahold of my thoughts. It simply allows me to breathe in fresh oxygen and free myself from distractions that may get in my way. Recently I have gotten into meditating… after years of trying to meditate in a big group setting with no success, I have finally conquered it on my own. Meditation doesn't come naturally for most, so keep trying. To get to this point, I simply google a five minute guided meditation, lie down on the carpet in my living room or on my bed, and go for it. It is the best! Try it and take time to free your mental distractions and let your thoughts flow.

3. Device Distraction

After a busy, distracting day, we frequently pursue more distraction by watching television, being on our phones or iPads, and playing video games. Often, I will notice people when they are standing in a line; bored, they absorb themselves in their phones to distract them from the discomfort of waiting. Sometimes I will even see couples out for a dinner together, yet both are on their phones (finding more connection through social media than with their own spouse who is sitting right in front of them). I once had a family in my office and they mentioned that they give their daughter her iPad when they go out for dinner, to distract her so they can sit longer and have an adult conversation!

Really? I suggested to the mom that they leave their daughter at home with a sitter, and she said, "But then we wouldn't spend time with her, and we want to take her to dinner with us."

I said, "Well, no time is spent with your little one when she is on her iPad." Ohhh...she thought. I have recently seen families out for dinner where the little one is watching a full length movie while they are eating. My daughters and I love going for sushi, and my youngest, who was six at the time, pointed out a mom and her four children waiting for their meal. For the entire lunch hour, they were all eating and texting. Seriously bizarre to me. My daughter still brings up that family we saw that day by saying, "remember that family mommy"?

When you sit and really think about why you are eating a meal together...is it really just for nourishment, or is this the time you would like to connect with your children and/or your spouse, who you haven't seen all day? I encourage you to make a conscious effort to keep your phone at home when you go out together, or keep it in your purse on silent so it is out of sight and out of sound. Stay engaged...allow yourself to experience boredom when you stand in a line-up and let your thoughts naturally flow into your mind. You may be surprised by what is really going on inside. You will also be amazed at what you notice and the connections you begin to make.

4. Substance/Food Distraction

We are notorious for waking ourselves up, or should I say warming ourselves up, for the day with caffeine. Clients often declare this as the best part of their day. Caffeine gives us a natural boost for the day. It makes us alert and keeps us strong and running so we can tackle our day. And for those of us operating on very little sleep, this spike of caffeine gives a fantastic release of adrenaline to get us through the day. At the end of the day, we are notorious for cooling ourselves off with beer, wine or mixed drinks. These beverages lower the heightened adrenaline, taking it down from the chaotic go-go pace to a calm, slowed down and mellow pace. Alcohol and caffeine are great masks for how we really feel. They act as distractions from what our body needs. Be aware of your patterns. Are you stressed out at the end of the day? Are you grabbing for alcohol to relax you in the evenings? And in the mornings, are you so tired that caffeine helps to perk you up and get you going?

Our food distractions cause us to eat regardless of whether we are full or hungry. So often, people are eating because they have to, and they don't feel the hunger pangs. We use food to distract us. When we are sad, depressed, or have had a bad day, food can act as a shield or mask for how we are actually feeling. The distraction causes some of us to make poor food choices and overeat without thinking about it, or for some of us, to not eat at all. Some of us distract ourselves with a number on the scale to guide us toward whether to eat or not. We use bribes, rewards, and guilt to distract from what our body really needs.

5. Spending Distraction

How many of you have distracted yourselves by overspending? We go on a shopping spree to bring some form of happiness into our lives. Some people get a rush over material things and attachments that mask and protect them, and in turn, distract them from what is really going on.

6. Social Media Distraction

How disconnected have we become from having real live face to face conversations with our friends and family? With one simple click on Facebook and within minutes you can be completely connected to your friends and acquaintances. You know who has had surgery, a baby, who's sick and who has received an award to name a few. With smiley faces, high fives, hearts and hands pressed together in Namaste, there is something great about this as well as thin and undigested. This accessibility and easiness of knowing it all is a great way to stay connected in an increasingly busy world, but it can also lack value, sincerity and human connection. I have been to parties and outings where the people I am with are taking pictures, tagging, posting and updating their status minute by minute and within mid conversation to keep their world connected. Where is the secret of calling someone up to ask how they have been?

Distractions that take us away from this world come in all different guises, from being on our phones, devices, and video games, to having the television on like a constant light in the home. Loud music, dish cleaning during meal time, family members eating at various times or getting up and down from the table constantly during a meal, are all forms of distractions. Distractions can be seen in the form of bribes, negotiations, and a reward system at the table. It can also be seen when children are fooling around at mealtime. Distraction comes from the busyness of life, from the stress of life. Our scattered minds distract us. Feeling ill or constantly having something wrong with us is a distraction too. It is crazy how being too busy is the current universally accepted excuse. I know I used to use it. Being busy gave me a sense of purpose and belonging in a world that accepts busy. Are you busy?

Do you like the distraction, are you procrastinating, or are you scattering your life with mindless stuff? Maybe you are afraid to say no?

Today for example, at my stepson's hockey game recently, I overheard the crowd cheering for one boy named Noah to get a goal. I was wondering why they were so excited as a group of adults to see this little man get a goal. Well, I soon figured it out; Noah's parents were paying him fifty dollars if he got a goal this game...which he did, of course; his first goal that season. Now why were the parents paying him? Was Noah motivated by the money to get the goal? Was he bribed to get the goal so his parents could feel a sense of joy and excitement watching him score? What was it? Just last week at my daughter's soccer game, I also overheard a little guy telling his dad that after the game, he gets six dollars, I guess a bribe for winning the soccer game. I thought, are you kidding me? Why the bribes and rewards? Why can't children just go out and have fun without the pressure to succeed? With this type of bribe and reward system, do children ever experience the pure thrill and satisfaction of just pushing themselves to score because they want to? Because they want to feel the pure satisfaction and rush that comes with achieving something on their own? To score so they can experience the amazing thrill it brings to them, to their team, and to their parents watching?

What do all of these distractions do to families?

They in fact cause us to drift away from connecting with our spouses and children. Distractions occupy your mind and take up space from just simply being and simply noticing.

Take this example; I had a lady in my office the other day who could not get her son to eat anything beyond chicken fingers, grilled cheese, and fries. In further discussion, we determined there were many distractions in their lives. One was the need for her husband and herself to connect with each other; so they used table time to have serious adult conversations, such as about bills. Secondly, they were distracting their little boy with the television or iPad, because that was the only way he would eat. The mom further mentioned that he immersed himself in the television so more spoonfuls of food could be consumed.

In another family scenario, a mother noticed her children didn't want to come to the table because their television show was starting or they needed to get back to their Xbox to play with their friends on line. She couldn't understand why her kids wouldn't eat and were constantly being pulled away from the table, until I brought to her attention the distractions her household was supporting.

Another example is the parent getting ready to feed their infant veggies for the first time. They set up the high chair and soon discover the only thing that works to get their child to eat is the television, cheerios on their tray, airplane sounds, cheering when the food goes in, and clapping. Toys and rattles are also used to keep the baby distracted from how much they are eating, what they are eating, and whether they are hungry or full. Furthermore, for most families, feeding an infant is a huge chore, so often the baby is fed away from the dinner table and away from meal time with the rest of the family. "Let's feed the baby first and then we will eat," is a common theme in families.

So what is really going on? Distractions stop us from feeling and connecting as a family. When we are distracted, we have no idea if the food even tastes good. We eat regardless of whether we are hungry or full. When distracted, we can eat without even acknowledging flavor. Take movie popcorn, for example. A large bag of popcorn can be completely finished during the movie, without even a thought to whether the popcorn tasted good or not or if you were hungry for more. Many people feel disgusting after eating movie popcorn. And the movie (we can blame it for this one) was distracting us the whole time from the hand in the bag, then in mouth motion. Autopilot, here we come.

So I need you to un-distract yourself first so you can begin to understand how distracted you and your children really are. Wake up and smell the roses! Have you ever simply sat in a chair and just let your mind wander, wander to what is outside, to the noises of the wind, to the sounds in your head?

Put down your phone, get off your computers, and turn off the noise of the television. Get rid of the news or the music in the background and just simply be present in the moment. What does your house smell like? What does your daughter look like? What is she saying to you? Did she call your name once or did she call your name three or four times to get your attention? How does it feel when she hugs you? Is she constantly acting out so you will notice her? Take this journey with me and let go of distraction. It takes practice, but with each opportunity for practice, you will become more aware, feel more, listen better, and begin to make life changing connections with your family that begin at the hub of the table!

6 BE PRESENT

As you let go of distraction, you will begin to focus on what it feels like to be present. When you take away devices, phones, televisions, and the scattered thoughts in your head, you will begin to wake up to what is happening around you. Take deeper breaths, listen to your body, and experience how you have the capability to take it all in. You will quickly become a great observer of things. An observer of what is really happening around you and within you.

Notice dimples on the knuckles of your child's hands (I love those), or freckles in new places. Listen to what your children are saying with the sweet, nonjudgmental, and innocent words they use to tell a story. Notice how you have the mental capacity to focus on a conversation and play games with your children. Be aware of how you are more able to listen to what your spouse has to say too.

Just the other day, for the first time ever, I went to the mall and instead of frantically shopping for something I had to pick up (I am not a big mall fan, although my daughter wishes I was) I decided to grab a cup of tea, a turkey wrap, and sit on one of those comfy seats smack dab in the middle of the mall. I decided for the first time ever to embrace the mall experience. Usually I am in and out of the mall within twenty minutes. I park at the closest space to the entrance. My mom taught me this parking technique. It felt like we would drive around for hours to find a spot as close to the entrance of the mall as possible. My grandma, when she was with us, used to pray for a close parking space and asked everyone in the car to pray with her. I did of course; there was really no way out of it. I actually closed my eyes and prayed to God that a parking spot would open up so I could be spared the craziness of finding a spot closest to the mall. And for some reason praying actually made a space appear. When we didn't seem to get one, my grandmother would always pipe in, "Somebody isn't praying." So I would pray harder. And, voila, we always got one. I guess the longer you wait and the more you pray, something will eventually come to you. Anyway, I am getting off track here; I have adopted the close to the entrance parking spot technique now. I enter the mall and go right for the directory. I find my store, grab what I need, and leave. But on this particular day, I instead grabbed lunch and sat smack dab in the middle of the mall. After I ate my lunch, I decided to hang out longer and just BREATHE and BE PRESENT in that moment. As I sat watching people rushing through the mall, I observed so much. I let my mind drift in and out, and deeper into relaxation. I was simply feeling, enjoying, and embracing. I had honored myself with the time to sit, relax, and let it go. At that moment, I could understand why people enjoyed simply sitting in the mall and watching the crowds go by. As crazy as it sounds, I felt free to just stop, do nothing, and be alone. What a fantastic feeling, in a place I used to avoid so much. The time passed, and I actually had to push myself to get up and continue on with the hustle and bustle of the shopping experience.

The dictionary defines being present as the period of time occurring right now. How many times do you stop and wonder where the day went? Or wonder, "What did I eat today, what did I do this past week?" For example, this year, winter was extraordinarily cold, and by March, after many snowfalls, I just could not wait for the warmer weather to come. By doing this, I wished away the last few weeks of the gorgeous spring weather we had without being aware of it. Suddenly, it was the end of April and May was just around the corner.

When we are present, time slows down. We know what we did that day and we begin to develop memories associated with our feelings. When we continue to wish for something more or something better, we lose sight of what we have, where we are, and how beautiful the fresh air feels. When we live without actually being present, we simply do not exist. We flutter through the day, masking, distracting, and protecting our true selves; and we lose awareness of the sounds of birds chirping, the wind in our ears, the little voice our child uses when they talk to us, or the little hands that touch us to find a connection.

I recently attended a women's recharge group, and one of the questions presented to me was, "If you could go anywhere or do anything that would bring you the most peace, what would it be? My answer came to me so quickly; it is lying on a blanket on a warm day, looking up into the blue sky, and just simply watching the clouds roll by. I love watching the clouds and the different pictures they create. I still recall the energy it brought me as a child. Through this experience, I can really be present with the cloud shapes and the amazing blue tones of the sky. Everything else around me is lost somehow, and as long as I look up, it is just me, the sky and the cool energy I get from it.

When we are present, we can see and feel so much. It is amazing what our bodies can actually tell us. My body is able to shout out to me when something I am doing doesn't fit with what I want or need. The shout outs come loud and strong when something I am doing, seeing, or hearing doesn't fit with my core value system. Something inside me says, STOP, WAIT, WHAT is this, BE CAUTIOUS. I don't even need to know really what my value system is; it is innate—in me and in all of us. So when something is off kilter, my body will tell me. I will hear things such as, "Get out, not good, move away," or "This situation, place, or person doesn't fit with you." My stomach will tell me this with a stomach ache and a thick, heavy head.

When you stop and think about it, the fact that when you are present, your body can actually tell you what is right for you and what is not right for you, is wild. And I can tell you, we all have this mechanism. This mechanism is so loud and strong, that for years, I would just distract myself. I would use tactics or make excuses to ignore how I felt, and then I would simply move on, pushing forward. I felt unbalanced, scattered, and stressed as I persevered through my day without presence of mind, body, or spirit continuing my super-busy schedule of things to do. I indicated this in my first chapter and in my first marriage. Just as with food and your tummy, where some foods work for you and others foods do not, situations, thoughts, and experiences have similar effects. Take the example of a child eating alone at the table while others are frantically on their devices, watching television, cleaning up, or running out the door. This leaves the child feeling lonely, unvalued or unwanted. And does that child want to eat their food with that feeling? Does their stomach hurt? Do they now feel full? Does their body tell them this situation does not feel good?

Or take the family who argues and yells at the table; does this feel comfortable and safe for the child to eat at the table. Are they still hungry? Or is their body telling them they need out? Consider the lady who comes home from work, and after eating dinner, sits on the couch and starts demolishing a bag of chips until they are gone. When she is done, she feels guilty, regrets it, and sometimes feels badly about herself. Why? Because she wasn't present when she did this, she wasn't feeling or listening to what her body needed. She simply ate all those chips out of habit, or based on a reward system. Bad day at work equals rewards with bad food when I get home. And we wonder why so many families can't get their children to eat. Just stop, lose the distraction, simplify your life, and be present.

Consider a family who eats together, shares laughs, and nourishes positive loving relationships at the table, where there is no judgment of how much you ate, how little you are, or what you ate. This allows those at the table to feel safe, present, and happy as they eat and nourish their bodies. Bribes, negotiations, rewards, and punishments are gone at their table.

When you stop and listen and you are present in a situation that doesn't sit well with you, where do you feel this in your body? Some feel it in their head (they get a headache), back pain, shoulder pain, they may rage or get upset. Some feel it in their chest. You may feel this when you walk into a store that doesn't feel good to you, or when you walk into a party or a group of people who don't fit well with you. Connect with this and give yourself some time to understand what your body is telling you. The stomach ache may not be due to the food you ate.

We are able to walk around with our amazing body every day and have it tell us what is good for us or what is not good for us. It is able to shut down those nonproductive voices in our head and simply say, "Yes, this is good for me," or "NO, this is not good for me."

Being present while we eat is so important. Are you full or are you hungry? What does your body want to eat? Are you craving? Are you tired? Is your body crying out for you to slow down? Are you sick or are you well? Most people have a difficult time with this. We are programmed to be ALL GOOD. Busy is the new norm. So the busier you are, the more valued you are as a person to some people. Or the busier you are, the more successful you must be, too. So we keep going so we can stop listening, eventually numbing ourselves of feelings. We move further and further away from our situation and the present place. We rush through life and never stop to consider what out body wants, what our body needs, or what our body is telling us. I teach clients that tummy aches, headaches, aches across the shoulders, high blood pressure, indigestion, overeating, emotional eating, under-eating, eczema, insomnia, burning eyes, and fungus in the toe nails, to name just a few, are all signs the body is trying to tell you something. When we just stop, breathe, and are present, we give our body a chance to be heard. When we listen, we are able to help our body before these aches and pains manifest in deeper health issues. We can teach children to do the same. Listen to your children when they have a tummy ache. For my daughter, a tummy ache and a headache are signs of anxiety and worry. It's probably much the same with adults, except we have been taught to suck it up, take a Tylenol or a Tums, and get on with our day. Actually listening to your children with empathy and being present in their shoes, asking them what is wrong, why do they think they have a tummy ache, or why do they have a headache, will help them to be more present and teach them to listen to what their body has to say. I noticed this recently in my youngest. If I was off or rushed, she would get a tummy ache. "My tummy hurts," she would say. And guess what? Her tummy did hurt. Her tummy was saying this pace of life doesn't work for me, or this pace of life doesn't sit well with me. As a mom, if I had said, "You are fine," and pushed along, she would bury how she was feeling and stop listening to those cues. Instead, stopping and asking what is wrong, slowing down, and offering a warm embrace helps the sore tummy and gets to the root of the problem.

I remember as a child, I would often get sharp tummy pains that would last for hours. Now looking back with the wisdom of my years, I see it was my body's way of telling me something was wrong. I would often have sleepless nights, too. I ignored it...moved on and got up for school the next day. Pushing through, keeping busy, and taking little time to stop and be present.

What I am getting at here is that when we as parents learn to live in the present moment, we can lead by example, so our children can learn to do the same too. We can stop the cycle of moving fast, pushing feelings away, and adding more distractions to our lives to mask the present moment. We can, in fact, break the cycle and begin to develop conscious children who know when they are full and when they are hungry. A child who knows what they want and what feels good. Who is able to sit without distraction and enjoy and embrace their surroundings. Isn't that what we want our children to be? A child who grows up without fear of peer pressure; a child who is definite about who they want to hang out with and what they want to do when they get older. This programming is within all of us. We all have the power to be present and listen to our bodies.

So how do you get to this PRESENT place? It is much easier to be present when you let go of distraction. Begin with a conscious practice. You really need to work at it to find success here. There will be days you fall back into your distracted, busy patterns, but there will be many days that are fantastic, too. I consciously have to tell myself this is my time to be with my children or to be with my spouse, and my text messages and e-mails can be put on hold until later. Often, my mind will drift away, and then I will bring my focus back to the present—back to pushing my daughter on the swing or having a conversation with my children in the car. Amazing how you can multitask in your mind to be having a conversation while thinking about what you are going to make for dinner. So often I will need to shut the dinner stuff down to be fully present with my daughter and her conversation. It takes practice. And especially because these little children of ours grow up so fast, you really do not want to miss any moments of their life. When I go out to the park for a walk, I leave my phone at home. I have phone time after the children go to bed. Or I schedule phone time so the family knows I will be distracted for a while at that time. I sometimes catch myself with my phone, so I have my children call me out on it. I ask them to tell me when they catch me sneaking in a text...I am so unconscious about it sometimes, so they help me be aware of it. Through practice, you can make it perfect, and you can actually begin to be OK without distractions.

Take a breath, pause, breathe again, and stop. Stop, observe, and listen to take in and feel all of the moments your life has to offer!

7 THE BIG DECISION

Starting a family was one of the biggest and most memorable events of my life. With so many discussions over common questions such as can we afford this, are we ready to commit to this, and how will this new bundle of joy fit into our lives, the decision to start trying to have a baby is one thing, but for all of us who have had children, when the baby actually arrives, it is absolutely another thing. There is no other way to slice it. The newborn is life altering in every way. My children have entirely changed my life. They will take over your life and run it, if you let them. At times, I would look at my little screaming bundle of joy in the wee hours of the night and think, "What I have done? Take this baby back to where it came from!"

Babies bring everything from interrupted schedules

and loss of sleep, to piles of laundry and a tummy that wants to be fed six to eight times every day. From potty training to completely living on demand, in fight or flight, parents need to be ready for anything. We strive as parents to be the rock for our children, trying to be everything to them all of the time. And as they get older, we drive them for the one hundredth time to music lessons and soccer practice. Then teenage years hit, with new schedules and routines. These teens no longer have a bedtime, and they tend to think they know what's best for them now. They don't need moms and dads; they just need their money (hahaha). Your teenage "baby" likes to spend most of their time socializing with friends and hibernating in their room. They have different social schedules that allow for this. They learn to drive (your car), get braces, and need help with post secondary education. They move in, move out, and then move back in again. The decision to have a family is a major commitment, and one of the hardest jobs in town. There is no play book or job description that fits any child. This is a commitment that is learned as you go, and is the only job where there is no pay and you are on call twenty-four hours a day.

Now, with the life changing events a baby can bring and the huge responsibility that goes along with it, infants, children, and teenagers do bring something to your life. Although they feel like they are takers, they are actually givers. And for each parent, this represents something different. For me, they are a complete miracle and a blessing. Their little fingers, their little toes, their perfect cry. It is unbelievable we can make these creations. The love you see in your baby's eyes as they look up at you when you hold them, hug them, and kiss them. The smile and pure excitement they give you when you say good morning to them and open your arms to get them out of their crib. The joy they bring to you when they ask you questions, ask you to teach them new words, or just want to hold your hand. Their contagious giggle when you kiss, hug them and do doggy sniffles in their ear. Their sponge-like ability to absorb everything you say and do. They ask you questions, and believe you and all of your wisdom. They follow you around, want to be picked up, played with, and listened to. Children look up to you for guidance, support, and reassurance that they are doing the right thing.

The other day, while driving, I reached my hand toward the back seat of my car where my six-year-old daughter was sitting, and I felt something wet hit my palm. Because I was driving, I could not see what she was doing behind me, I could only feel. I asked, "Did you kiss my hand?" And she said, "YES!" and started giggling profusely. I said, "That was so nice!" Because I acknowledged how nice her actions were, and she could see how they made me feel, she continued to kiss my hand with big kissing noises when I reached back. With each kiss, her giggle became louder and my smile became wider, until we were both laughing together. The feeling of giving and receiving was amazing for both of us to share. All parents should experience the pure joy children give to us in some way or another.

The Journey Begins

Now, let's talk about this bundle of joy in the womb. From the moment you find out you are pregnant, the fun appointments begin. With each checkup, you are measured, weighed, and assessed. Your life becomes all about getting your little embryo to fruition, and for those of us who don't conceive right away, the journey to pregnancy can look far different from the one-shot deal some couples are blessed with.

Regardless of how long it took to get to pregnancy, once you've told everyone you're expecting, friends and family begin guessing how big your baby is going to be based on how your belly is growing. Sometimes weight contests at work and at baby showers take place. The weight of the newborn baby is a big deal during this very exciting time. You have appointment after appointment, weigh-ins, and constant monitoring, and finally, your baby arrives after what feels like an eternity. You announce whether you had a boy or a girl and how much your baby weighed. Years later, most moms can remember how big their baby was when they were born. After delivery, your baby continues to be assessed, examined, and weighed to be sure they are growing "properly." In other words, not just growing, but growing according to standards set by government statistics. Moms and dads start to become nervous and perhaps even panicked when their baby is off the growth chart or not on the growth chart. They talk in percentiles, and at just a few months old, parents know exactly what category their baby is in. Now the comparison to other babies begins. We think making sure our baby grows up to standards is a God-given right! It has been ingrained in us. Taking on this responsibility can be very overwhelming for most parents. Think about it. What happens if your baby is growing beneath standards (smaller than average), how does that make you feel? Or if your baby is growing above standards (bigger than average)? How does that feel to you?

I remember with my firstborn, I lived at the breastfeeding clinic. I thought things were going pretty good when she was born. I was soon mistaken. After delivery, we stayed in the hospital for a little less than twenty-four hours (this is the norm from where I am from). I made a decision to try breastfeeding. During our time in the hospital, nobody had time to check on how my daughter was latching or feeding. When I left the hospital, I was going on day six before I saw my GP for the first time. After weighing my new bundle of exhaustion, my doctor said, "She has lost too much weight, please go straight to the maternity ward at the hospital; I will call and tell them to expect you. Your daughter needs to be assessed," she continued. UGH, there is that darn word again. What does this mean, I wondered? Is my baby OK? Is something wrong? What did I do? I thought everything was going well. With that, I bundled my newborn daughter up in a blanket, left my car where it was in the parking lot by the doctor's office, and walked with her in my arms down the street to the hospital, tears rolling down my face. My hormones really were getting the best of me at the time. Lack of sleep and a baby who wasn't feeding is a combination for disaster (all moms can vouch for this). I am sorry, but there is nothing natural about "the latch." My nipples were burning, bruised, and battered! I ended up in the breastfeeding clinic at the hospital, where I stripped my baby girl down and she was weighed. I nursed her and she was weighed again, naked and cold! They told me she wasn't getting enough milk. So back on my breast my daughter had to go for more milk. I remember cringing in tingling pain as she latched. I felt like giving up as warm tears continued to trickle down my cheek. All I did was feed my baby. That was all I did! My new life was all about breastfeeding, making sure she was getting enough, and scheduling in pumping between feedings. It was exhausting. I often asked myself what the heck I was doing. When I sought advice, everyone's answer was "You are doing great." But I didn't feel that way at all. I guess you can never truly prepare yourself for the changes in your own body and then the changes in your own life with raising a baby. Nobody said to just give her formula. I was already feeling torn trying to get food into this tiny baby of mine. It was a chore. The breastfeeding clinic and the constant monitoring felt like the only way to get through this rough patch, so I just went with the flow. There was nothing natural about this and my daughter suddenly wasn't in control of how much she was eating. I was in control of how much, and ultimately, the breastfeeding clinic was, too. And this was all based on a growth chart and a scale. I ended up going every day, renting the electric pump from the nurses' station. Breastfeeding by day and pumping by night. Ohh what fun! I remember after six weeks they told me I could not come back. They said I was done. I thought, Ohh no. How am I ever going to trust that my baby is eating enough and growing?

And this is how it all begins for most parents. The control sets in for parents with the journey of making sure their baby is eating enough, eating the right things, and growing enough—not too much and not too little. What would happen if we just let all of that go to fate? To have faith in the fact that our bodies grew a beautiful healthy baby in nine months of which we had no control, we just trusted. To have faith that now that our baby is out in the world, they have the instincts to know when they are hungry and when they are full. To trust that their bodies know when to store food for upcoming growth and when to let it all go again.

I was back to work six weeks postpartum and completed breastfeeding by six months. I wish I had let the guilt of it all go sooner. I was torn between breastfeeding my baby and formula feeding. Well, not initially, when it was a no brainer for me that I was going to breastfeed. But when it actually all came to fruition, it was much harder than I had anticipated. The latch, the screaming baby for food when there wasn't any, and the exhaustion I felt with each feeding—I knew something was wrong. I remember at every mom's group, it was always a topic of discussion with all the other moms. You knew exactly who in the group were breast feeders and who were bottle feeders. There was a stigma attached to bottle feeding moms.

When my second daughter was born, it was much easier, and I just realized what worked best for me and our family was the right decision. I had a lactation consultant who worked with me in the clinic I owned at the time, and because I had some health issues going on in my family, with being back to work a week after my daughter was born, I made a decision to breast and bottle feed in combination. It was a brilliant idea for me and one I felt really comfortable with. It felt so liberating and perfect for our situation, and our daughter really took to this routine. I was able to breastfeed as often as I could and bottle feed when my daughter was left home with dad or nana so I could work. I vividly remember heating up a bottle for my daughter at my clinic and the lactation consultant jumping down my throat about bottle feeding versus breastfeeding. She was beside herself, and couldn't understand why I would do such a thing. I was very grateful she was so knowledgeable and that she cared so passionately for her role in helping moms, but it was also my decision and my baby, and the mixing of feeds worked for us. I couldn't help but feel that all of our problems with feeding our children in modern society are due to standards that are approved and accepted by others. Are you eating organic? Is your child drinking kale smoothies? Are you breastfeeding? Are you making your own baby food?

Through all of these judgments society puts on us, we are missing the biggest component—the connection between parents and children. We are forcing food into the forefront of this connection, to control a baby's first instinct to eat or not eat, and then we continue this pattern into toddlerhood and childhood. Think about this for a moment; the first thing a baby does when they are born is cry, and then they eat. At just seconds old, the newborn baby knows they are hungry. And with breastfeeding moms especially, we have no measurement of how much they are eating when our baby feeds. We just trust that when the baby pulls off the breast or pulls away from the nipple or the bottle, they are full and satisfied. A perfect cue that was developed by mother nature. And then it is amazing, every two and a half to three hours, like clockwork, the baby screams for more food. They know exactly when they are hungry and when they are full. This is AMAZING! God made these great creations, these little miracles; he made human beings with a mechanism to know when they want food and when they do not want food. Yeah, thank god! So why do we mess it all up? Why do we go in and forget this? We think our children have no idea when they are hungry and when they are full. In fact, we take this gift away from them. We numb it instead of embracing it. What a cool thing it is to be able to know exactly when you are hungry and exactly when you are full. In adulthood, we see so many who are not able to utilize the hunger/full mechanism because it has been dulled by so many years of weight loss program after weight loss program. The body just literally shuts that gift down. So in turn, we simply do not think children are capable to make the decision about how much fuel their body requires. How do we really know how much they need? If every baby grows on a different curve and every child continues to grow differently, we really have no idea what each individual person needs. We limit food or force feed, bribe, and offer rewards to get our children to eat more or less because we are so controlled by growth charts, scales, what we have learned and what others may think.

Food becomes very emotional. It is the first thing that we as humans know we need, and because we have triggers to know how much we need, it becomes a basic necessity that when tampered with or altered, can affect our emotional well-being and confidence. To be told you have had too much to eat or you need to eat more, to be bribed emotionally when a mother says "It will make me so happy if you ate two more bites," or when dad jumps up and down and hugs his child for finishing their dinner, or when a crying child is offered food to comfort her, all begin a process of emotional eating.

When parents lose the control of their children and begin to use food to negotiate a pattern for the day, they teach their children to stop listening to their body's cues and begin to follow the emotion of what mommy or daddy wants them to do.

They eat to receive more love and comfort from mom and dad (praise, hugs, and kisses when meals are eaten). Some parents even go so far as to punish their child if they don't eat or are not hungry...sounds crazy, doesn't it? Or some say things such as, "You will make mommy so happy if you eat five more bites." Or "It makes mommy so sad when you do not eat your dinner."

Do you see how food begins to control our child's emotional well-being? At first glance, these requests from parents seem to make common sense; simple pleas from parents to avoid temper tantrums and arguments. Make no mistake, this is a trap. Well intentioned parents trying to make mealtime work find themselves falling into negotiations that include bribes, rewards and consequences. Food is used as a power source to control instead of the source of nourishment that it was intended to be.

A child hears, "Mommy and daddy will love me more, give me hugs, or give me a treat if I eat" or "Mommy always smiles, appears happier and jumps for joy when I eat." These techniques disconnect children from knowing how much fuel their bodies need and how often they need that fuel. Food, and mealtime end up being all about control. This doesn't just create a negative relationship with food, it creates the foundation for a negative relationship between child and parent in all aspects of life.

Now as parents continue to negotiate when and how much food should be eaten, so many children go without when their parent is not around to help them eat. Take school for example, so many times I hear parents say their child will go all day without eating. Do you know why this is? Because mom or dad has always told this child when to eat and how much before they can get up and go again. They are programmed to listen to mom and dad's cues dictating when they should eat and how many more bites they need to take. I see children play while their parents chase them around to put a spoonful of food into their mouth. This is so disconnected from what our bodies need, want, and desire. Please don't get me wrong, this all comes from a loving place. A place where we want the best for our children, but we begin to quickly see that food has taken power over us, and the dynamic around the dinner table has shifted from a place of fun and connection to one of control, power, bribes, and rewards.

8 THE POWER OF THE BODY

How do you feel when I say every sperm and egg that unite to make up a healthy embryo has the same fighting chance as another embryo to have a metabolism that operates perfectly? A metabolism that tells the body when fuel is needed, and one that tells the body when enough fuel has been received. One that makes sure everything within the body is nourished properly, from the bones and muscles, to the hair, and down to the toes. A metabolism that balances hormones and manufacturers them in the liver properly. One that gets rid of toxins and fights disease. A metabolism that builds a healthy immune system, one that provides nutrients for healthy brain function and a metabolism that allows the body to survive optimally.

Every baby that is born, regardless of their size at

birth, has the same chance as the next baby to never have to diet, lose weight, or limit calories in any capacity for as long as they live. Pardon, you say? You heard me. Everyone should and could live free of ever having to diet again. Which means obesity issues would be gone and emotional eating would be over. This book was written to help one person at a time, one family, or one child. Every newborn baby has the same fighting chance to be a strong, vibrant, loved, accepted, grounded, and self-confident human being, and this all begins at the table.

You know when that child loses that fighting chance? The moment mom and dad begin to control how much food is right for their child. This is the absolute game changer. This is the exact point when things begin to change.

How many times have you noticed in your children that two to four months before a growth spurt, they eat nonstop? Nothing you give them satisfies them. If a parent was to use devastating comments to control their child's intake, saying things like "You've had too much," or heaven forbid, "You'll get fat if you eat more," their child's body would slow down its growth and development to a suboptimal level, often functioning at a survival level. When food is limited, the body holds food in reserves, for fear it may not have enough fuel for daily functioning. More often than I would like to see happen in my practice, parents look at the size of their child instead of truly understanding the day to day functions their child's body is handling on the inside to grow longer and stronger bones and muscles. To grow bigger eyes, nose, hands, feet and more red blood cells and to have enough fuel to take a child into puberty or get them through their day to day activities.

Often, bodies will hold onto nutrients and bulk up in anticipation for an upcoming growth spurt. During this time, the children who are being limited in their food intake may not grow healthy bodies. They may fail to grow a body that makes the call when nutrients are needed, rather than looking to an outside judge such as parents, who feel their child has had enough according to standards or comparisons to other children. Did you know that your body knows days before you do that a sickness is lingering? It gears up and tries to fight off the virus or infection before it takes over your body. It increases your body's core temperature by producing a fever to kill off the germs. If a body is functioning in survival mode (not receiving enough food or nutrients) already, it becomes quite difficult for it to have the energy to fight off infections or abnormal cells that float around our bodies on a daily basis. There is so much going on behind the scenes of our amazing bodies that we do not know about, just like a baby who cluster feeds during a growth spurt or begins to wake up in the middle of the night for more food when they were sleeping through the night previously. Have you ever wondered why in the past babies were given cereal when they were not sleeping well? Now we are told to wait until a certain age, holding off due to guidelines with the basis that starting cereal early will bring on food allergies. Whether it does or it doesn't, these growing babies require more fuel and are shouting out for it. Again, all babies are different, and each requires different amounts of food at different stages.

Why fiddle around with mother nature? Have you ever noticed how a baby gets enormous roll after roll in the inner thighs of their legs? Do you know why that is? This is storage for when they require the fuel for growth. Their body prepares itself well in advance before the growth happens. Think of how bodies grow and if a child expended as much energy as they put in, there would not be room to grow bigger bones, a bigger spine and a bigger skull, to name a few. If babies are meant to grow, then why are some babies bigger, with tons of loving rolls, and other babies are smaller? Both babies eat the same, but both grow and require energy in different ways. If the parent who had the roly poly baby limited food intake and began to change serving sizes, that baby might not grow and develop to their fullest potential. Brain function, bones, and muscles require fuel. Building our children up to create strong bones and allowing them to eat for growth is key for proper development in all areas of their life. We need to trust and let growth flow.

Children continue to grow until they are fourteen to seventeen years of age. Some start puberty as young as seven years old, and others start when they are sixteen. There is a huge discrepancy. So it is unfair to compare one child to another child as they are all so different in their development and the fuel requirements their body needs at every stage.

No longer can you look at a child and assume that because they are bigger than the rest of their peers, they are unhealthy or fed the wrong foods. Lots of healthy children have midsection weight gain before they grow taller, leaner, and stronger. And all children grow at different rates.

Another factor besides growth that we need to watch for is that when a parent with a larger child limits serving sizes and starts focusing on body size, their child grows up to struggle with weight, due to what they were told as a child. They do not grow to their full, healthy potential. As well, limiting food messes around with metabolism, so the body begins to learn at an early age to hold onto food and store it as it comes in limited doses. The other situation I see is the child who fears gaining weight (even for growth spurt purposes) because they have seen the struggles their mother or father have had with weight issues (counting calories, dieting, obsessive weighing, and over-exercising). Some parents will make comments such as, "I'd better not have any more," or "Why did I eat all of that?" or "I just ate way too much food," or "I think I have had enough." Like little sponges, children are constantly scanning, watching, and listening to their parents' comments and actions, and they begin to formulate their own guidelines around food and what is enough or too much for them, so the cycle continues. Take a moment to think about how food was presented to you as a child. Was it limiting? Was your mother checking her weight constantly or pushing food away from herself in fear another spoonful would cause the scale to change? Did your mom sneak chocolate into her bedroom to snack on or sit on the couch at the end of the day and binge eat? Did she use words such as fat and compare herself to others with a focus on body image?

These types of environments are cyclical and get passed down from generation to generation if the cycle isn't stopped. Doesn't it just make more sense knowing all that we know about how bodies grow, to allow our children to determine how much food they need? It is a huge relief for parents to know that our bodies are designed to be smart consumers, to know exactly how much fuel we require. So stop fiddling around and changing the mechanics of these amazing bodies. Stop comparing your child to another child, or yourself to someone else. Stop worrying about growth or what people may think. Let go of the fear of judgment if your child is smaller or larger than the child next door. Yes, worry does come from such a very loving place, but recognize that it can be a bad thing. Let go of the notion, that if you don't force a carrot down your child's throat or stop them from taking another bite, they will not grow. They will ☺.

9 EMOTIONAL ATTACHMENT

The outcome of force feeding and/or threatening a child over their eating is the child begins to eat because they have to, not because they want to, and they stop listening to their own body. The fear is that these children later develop struggles with weight gain and weight loss; priding themselves on body image to obtain a higher sense of self-worth. This is an epidemic.

Parents use food and table time as a vehicle to show their love and acceptance to their children, feeding their children whatever they want and offering rewards through food for good behavior. Gone are the days we would show our love through our actions and words. Parents are finding themselves saying things such as, "You won't grow if you don't eat," or "You will make mommy so happy if you eat," or "Mommy feels really sad that you didn't eat your dinner tonight." These words play huge roles in how food makes children feel and the emotional attachment that goes along with it. Sometimes I hear, "You only get dessert if you eat one more bite," or "No ice cream for you if you don't eat your dinner." This approach affects how we make connections with food and weight and the scenario of being good or bad based on what we eat. Why should foods be put into a hierarchy? We make ice cream seem better than broccoli—why? Because it works as a bribe. We punish our kids if they don't eat, or we sometimes yell at them. We find that this cyclical pattern is a tough one, and is difficult for parents to break. I am not bringing up these scenarios to make you feel guilty, but rather to offer you some insight on how our actions and words really affect our children.

I know that all you have done so far to feed your children comes from such a good place—a loving place as I have stated previously, because you love your children so very much! BUT, we can love differently, without using food as that vehicle. And when you take away food carrying loving control, children have an amazing relationship with their body image and will grow in a much stronger, more confident way. When mom and dad take those bribes, rewards, and punishments away and show their love through hugs and kisses, while keeping food on an equal hierarchy, it helps children develop positive attitudes and relationships toward food. It disconnects the emotional attachment to food and children begin to develop a positive self-image. Words such as, "I got a great mark on my report card so I deserve an ice cream cone" are crazy. Instead, use praise and acknowledgement of how proud you are of your children instead of food as the vehicle for reward. You can have an ice cream cone whenever you want. Not because you have been good. In adulthood, we eat a bag of chips in front of the TV because we think if we've had such a rough day, we deserve a bag of chips. Using food for comfort is where my term jail cell dieting falls into place. Until we break the emotional attachment to food, we will forever struggle with our weight as a society. So we are breaking this attachment today. When dessert is being served, everyone gets dessert, regardless of what they ate or did not eat or how well they behaved. Follow me here...

When the body doesn't get the appropriate amount of food at the time of asking, the body shifts its metabolism to a storage container for food and holds onto nutrients when they do finally come in. Often, children who are force fed become closet eaters, hide chocolate bars in their room, throw their lunch away at school, or shove food in their pockets to throw out when they get up from the table to use the washroom. These children fear they will not be the body type their parents want for them, or they stop eating to control something in their life. Chaotic, busy families, or families who scream and yell a lot, with domineering parenting, will often have a child who stops eating to exert control. These children and their parents use food as a source of power, "If you eat this, I will give you this." Or, "If you do not eat two more bites, you will not be able to go outside and play." Or, "If you don't eat your dinner, I will get very angry with you." Or, "It makes mommy so happy to see you eat," and she kisses and hugs her child because of it. Think about it! To a child, these words are powerful. The message they get is if I eat, I will make my mom happy, and she will show me she loves me more; if I don't eat, I will make my mom angry. And if I don't eat one day but then I eat the next day, I will have a mom who loves me the MOST.

Food really holds this much power? The child begins to formulate assumptions around eating or not eating and uses food as a power play when they say they don't like something, refuse to eat something they ate before, or have a tantrum because the food that is being served is something they do not like. The food may be touching another food on their plate, or they didn't get to sit in the seat they wanted to at the table. These are all power struggles where food is now connected to emotion, lending it a powerful significance. Are these scenarios ringing a bell for you?

Other examples are a child who needs to be spoon fed, sits on a parent's lap to eat, or gets up and down from the table constantly. This family endures a great deal of emotional power struggles with their children, and they tend to cave and simply feed the child what they like. These children can develop insecurities around food, and lose the understanding of what their body requires to grow. These children grow up with jaded views on portions and nutritious foods; and later in life, find they have trouble controlling their weight, resulting in yo-yo dieting, or my term, jail cell dieting (always stuck on a diet for fear they will gain weight). These children typically are emotional eaters and reward themselves with food when they have been good or have had a tough day. They see food as something they DESERVE instead of something their body NEEDS.

We are educated people, who realize all children grow at different paces. Some grow tall very quickly and others take time. The body needs to be prepared when the growth spurt is going to happen, or the body will scavenge the valuable nutrients and energy it needs from bone and muscle.

So here is what I say to you: It is so important to provide nutritious meals for your children. Let children eat freely, comfortably, and at their own pace. Allow your child to choose how much they would like to eat and avoid force feeding, bribing, rewarding, or telling them they will get fat if they eat something. Think of the words you are using and why you feel the way you do around this subject. So many parents struggle with their own body image which then trickles down to how their children feel about their own bodies. Please be sure you treat every child the same. Whether big, small, or growing. This is vitally important if children are to grow and develop positive self-esteem and self-worth in every aspect of their life. I cannot emphasize this enough.

Just yesterday after school, both my children were offered the same opportunity to snack on what they preferred. I stock my cupboards with healthy options (we will talk about these later) and it is at this time they have a choice of what they would like to snack on. My now seven-year-old (she just had a birthday, time flies) ate eight strawberries, two slices of organic raisin toast, half a cup of organic vanilla yogurt, and one homemade granola bar. Then she was ready to go off and play. She is hitting a growth spurt within the next few months, and this is her body's way of saying I need more fuel to accommodate this. You can't get money from a tree. Just like you can't make longer bones and stronger muscles from lack of food. I have been noticing she's been very hungry, and she will even amaze herself when she eats bigger portions or finishes everything on her plate. My eleven-year-old, on the other hand, is currently using her stored energy (she has been working hard building this up over the past two years) and is sprouting up like a bean pole. Yesterday, she opted to just have one slice of organic raisin toast for her snack after school, and today she chose not to have anything at all. Allowing my children to listen to their bodies and make the choice of how much fuel they need is the only way to feed children properly.

Here are three key points so far that I want you to work on:

Key #1:

Allow your child to decide whether they are hungry or full, and give them the choice of how much they would like to eat.

Key #2:

Provide nutrient dense options for all meals and snacks (let's face it; they get plenty of the other stuff at parties, school, and friends' houses). A sample list of snacks is provided in later chapter.

We as parents make the choice of what to provide, and your child chooses how much they would like to eat. Fair enough? Sounds easy, doesn't it?

Key #3:

Everyone in your household eats the same meal. No longer are mom or dad the third order cook. Cook one meal that the whole family will eat together, regardless of the likes or dislikes of the individuals.

Key number three is a very important rule. It is imperative that hotdogs, mac and cheese, and broccoli or fish are all on the same playing field. One is just as good or necessary as the other, so we get out of the reward system of junk food versus healthy food. Have you ever been to McDonald's and heard a parent bribe their child to eat two more bites of their chicken nugget before they can get up and play. Or how often have you seen parents chasing their child around McDonald's with a hamburger in their hand asking the child to take bites as they come down the Play land slide. What is the rationale here?

Now for the child who isn't eating. The one who refuses to eat needs the same rules. You may make excuses for them, in fear they will have a tantrum, saying, "They will never eat again if I serve them what the rest of us are eating." What you are really saying is, "They will never eat again if I serve them healthy foods." WRONG! I have been doing this for fifteen years, and I can promise you, your child will eat when left alone and able to make their own choice. I am offering you an easy step-by-step strategy that works. We will talk about this further in the upcoming chapters. So just hear me out for now as we continue to build this foundation together. The eating child (likes most things or is always hungry) and the non-eating child (likes few things or is never hungry) need to be offered nutrient dense meals where everyone is eating the same thing. They then can make the choice whether to eat or not to eat. It is very important you make the choice of what is being served and your child chooses if and how much they would like to eat. You both have two very defined roles.

We now know that forcing a child to eat doesn't work, bribing a child to eat doesn't work, and rewarding a child to eat doesn't work either. Well, let me rephrase that. These tactics work initially, but over the long term, they start to control the inner voice of the child's metabolism. Over the long run, it doesn't allow the child to listen to their own needs and grow and develop in a healthy, nourishing way. It also begins to develop those crazy emotional power struggles I spoke about earlier. Oddly enough, I just had a scenario at our house that relates to this, and I found myself getting ready to bribe, force, and punish to get my child to take her vitamin. I really want my eleven-year-old to start taking a vitamin. She has taken this in the past, but now I want to become more consistent with it, and make it part of our morning breakfast routine. I brought it out with her other supplements, and she immediately said, "Eww, I hate that one."

So I said, "It is just a vitamin, and you have had it before." She said, "It tastes funny and it is so big." She is right, it does taste funny and it is enormous. So I left the tablet out on the counter and told her she needed to have it before the end of the day. When dinnertime came that evening, I could feel my blood boiling. I was finding myself again forcing her to take it against her will, and the next day, when we did the supplement routine, she outright refused and said, "You can't force me to take it." It was at that moment that I made a decision. I could get very angry, begin a power struggle, take control and shove it down her throat with bribes, threats, and rewards, or I could agree she was right. I can't force her to take her supplement and I do want her to take control of her own body. So I let it go. And I will for a while. At least she is taking the other supplements freely, and she will take the one I want her to take in her own time, but I have to be good with the fact that it is her body and what she puts into her body is her choice. This is a hard concept as a parent. We think we have this control. But you know you can't force a lettuce leaf down your child's throat; it just won't go!

Below are some examples of the emotional power struggles food can have over us:

a)   Bribe

What is a bribe? If you have one more bite you can have some more pasta. Or if you finish your chicken you can go outside and play tonight, or you can stay up late tonight, or we can go to the movies, etc.

b) Reward

What is a reward? If you eat your dinner, then you can have dessert. If you do not eat your dinner, there is no dessert, or you can choose what you would like for dinner tomorrow night. A reward is also when a child gets a great mark on a project at school or has had dental work done for example, and they are now being shown congratulatory gestures through food.

c) Punishment

What is punishment? If you don't eat your dinner, I will be so angry at you. If you don't have three more bites, there is no TV tonight or your video games are taken away, or you will sit at the table until you finish everything on your plate.

d) Expressing Love Through Food

What is love through food? You make mommy so happy when you eat your dinner. Mommy needs to kiss and hug you all over for eating your dinner, you made mommy so proud. Mommy gets really sad when you don't eat. It makes me really angry when I make a meal for you and you do not eat. If you don't eat, you will not grow, or no more food because you have already had too much. Too much will make you fat.

Parents are at the root of the problem. We get worked up that our child may not eat, fearful they may not grow, so we resort to bribing, punishing, and rewarding for eating, which pushes our child further away from wanting to eat and further away from the safe family dinner table hub. It becomes a vicious cycle that we get wrapped up in. These children become picky eaters who like junk food and they hide and eat chocolate bars in their room to make up for the lost calories, leading to binge eating. Lots of parents will cater to these children and feed them only what they like to stop the table wars and feeding struggles and get them to at least eat something.

I would like to conclude this chapter with reiterating the three Golden Keys I discussed earlier, as well as add in a fourth Key I need you to begin to implement in your family. You may find as you implement these that some meals go great and others take you back to where you were before you got here. With practice and perseverance, I promise you will begin to master these four Golden Keys:

1. Provide a variety of nutrient dense snacks and meals for your children (a list of examples is provided).

2. Everyone at the table needs to be eating the same meal. So if hot dogs are served for dinner, you need to be sure you are also eating hot dogs along with your children. No longer is there a kids' menu and

adults' menu in your household. The exception here is when you are at a restaurant. Each family member can choose what they would like at a restaurant. This is important! Avoid telling your child what they should have and just allow them the choice. You may direct them to the kids' menu or the adult menu, depending on their age, but let them make the decision!

3. Your children have the choice whether they eat what is being served and how much they eat of it. They also have the choice to have second or third helpings if they so choose.

4. The fourth key is: take bribes, treats, rewards, and punishment away for good.

Now that seems all fine and dandy. Easy for me to sit here and write this to you. But when you actually go ahead and implement these Golden Keys, you will find that your children will act out. Tantrums, talking back, and causing a scene at the table are just a few examples. So in the next couple of chapters, I have outlined in more detail how to implement these four Golden Keys at each step and stage of your child's development. So hang tight as I begin to take you on a more detailed journey of how to feed your family, bring back the Family Table that pulls a disconnected family back to connection, and puts a stop to the emotional eating cycle.

10 INFANCY TO ADULTHOOD

The Baby and the Table

Very soon after a baby is born, we can see that a baby knows exactly how much food they need. It still astonishes me how smart the human body is at just a few minutes old. Isn't it incredible when you actually stop and think about it? A little peanut growing inside you (well that's amazing in itself), comes out into this world and already has the program hooked up that tells them to eat when they are hungry and to stop eating when they are full. Can somebody tell me where this program went as we got older? I recently visited with a mom on our street who just had a precious baby girl, and when I asked her how things were going in her first couple of weeks, she said, "I don't have to do anything, I just provide and my baby does all the rest." That is exactly right, we provide and babies eat what they need to fuel their bodies. The rest takes care of itself. Nutrients are delivered when needed, and growth happens when it is supposed to happen.

Just recently, I went to visit this little bundle again, and she seemed to want to cluster feed...she was tired and hungry all in one combination. After her feeding, I got a chance to cuddle her with her soother to pacify her, and she slowly drifted off to sleep. But not for long! She opened her eyes at the noise of children and was back to wanting to be fed again. She knew she needed more...and with another feeding, she was in lala land and off to sleep; nothing would wake her then.

How did we lose this mechanism in adulthood? As a society, we have gotten lured into yo-yo dieting and calorie counting cycles, and ignoring signs of hunger, with our day being valued by the number on the scale or how our clothes fit on our body. The scale has become our oracle to tell us whether we have been good or bad. Is this seriously what it has come down to? If your weight is up, you have been bad, and if your weight is down, you have been good. Please tell me this isn't true. Guess what—it is true! I see client after client come into my office saying they use the scale so they can stay on track with their weight. When they are up, it puts them in an emotional state of mayhem. Forming all sorts of guilty feelings and thoughts surrounding a lack of self-worth that forces them to eat to lose weight or pushes them to starve themselves to lose weight, because they have been so bad—or at least that is what the scale tells them.

This emotional eating rollercoaster has gotten the better of us. We no longer know when we are hungry or full, and if we are hungry, we feel guilty for feeling that way. Does this sound familiar? Well if it sounds familiar to you, it is also sounding familiar to your children. They are a product of what is becoming an emotional eating epidemic. As a society, we have lost the ability to feel good inside, so instead we use the scale, that ridiculous number, to tell us how we will feel each day. Here me out as I continue to explain where all of this comes from.

Newborn babies have zero pickiness in their soul; feed me breast milk if that's your decision, mom, or feed me formula; mom you choose, I'm cool with whatever. Do you get how simple this is so far? Are you seeing the pattern?...Mom you choose. Keep following me here. There is nothing picky about that. Just feed me what you've got and I will take it...oh, and thank you very much! Like clockwork, every two to three hours, the newborn baby squirms and cries for more food. Their stomach has a mechanism to tell the brain more fuel is needed here for proper growth and development. And that message stays with us for the rest of our lives. Can you hear it? Does your body tell you when you are hungry and when you are full? Does it really stop you in your tracks to eat your meals and your snacks in between meals? Well if it doesn't now, it used to, once upon a time long ago. That message in babies is so profound, the baby can end up screaming if they are left too long before being fed. I always see this at the grocery store. I was that mom, the mom who pushed the envelope to do one more errand before stopping to feed my daughter. The timer was on and I was always stuck in the checkout line behind a big grocery order in front of me with a few price checks and unscannable items in between, pacifying my daughter and wondering if I would be able to make it home before she exploded. Well in all seriousness, my daughter wouldn't explode, her basic need just would not be met when she needed it to be—yikes! That noise they produce is so demanding. A baby is sleeping soundly and then, BOOM, they are awake and hungry.

I teach this stuff, and every day I am in awe at how the human body works. The human body can stir that baby in the blink of an eye to eat. And what is even greater is that baby knows how much they want once they get it. A breastfeeding mom has no idea how much milk their baby is receiving. They simply trust the baby knows how much they need. What an amazing concept. The mom provides, and the baby controls whether they eat and how much they eat. This is so cool! And this is so easy! Stay with me here. It is truly that simple, and it all stems from these amazing bodies we carry around with us everywhere; they know what we need. But at some point, this all becomes a bit more complicated. It is easy for me to say babies like breast milk or formula, and they know when they are hungry and how much they need; BUT when more foods are introduced, and a baby's feeding requirements change due to growth, this feeding frenzy becomes a bit more intense.

Babies become interested in human food when they begin to eye your meal. They move their hands and feet in excitement, and their eyes watch your every move as you scoop a piece of broccoli from your plate to your mouth. That's when you know your baby is ready for the good stuff. Some of us decide to feed our baby directly from the table. This is a fantastic approach and one I highly recommend. This is called baby-led weaning. This is not about weaning baby off milk, but rather about weaning baby onto solid foods. Babies are then encouraged to eat what the rest of the family is eating This approach encourages the baby to join the family at meal times, getting the infant sitting around the table, seeing and experiencing the family together while self feeding appropriate finger foods. Remember this is an exploration of food at this stage and not how the infant will sustain themself. With this approach, on their own the infant gets to choose what they would like to eat off of their high chair tray. They choose how much and how quickly they would like to eat as well. This approach follows the exact same philosophy the child was born with. My mom chooses breast milk or formula (what is being served) and I get to choose how much I would like to eat. Through this approach, parents use their discretion and cut food into very small pieces that their baby can pick up, gum around in their mouth, and swallow. If cereal is being introduced, parents can help to spoon feed their baby until their baby is ready to experiment with the spoon themselves. This approach gets messy, but is the finest way a child can explore.

Let's visualize the opposite approach, where the baby is being spoon fed some jarred/homemade concoction that is different from what the rest of the family is eating. They are now not free to explore, and they tend to not be included around the family table. Remember the baby was eyeballing and interested in what you were eating initially, and this is why we brought them to the table to explore. With the jarred/homemade baby food scenario, the baby is spoon fed at a pace that suits the parent, as well as in amounts the parent feels is appropriate for baby. This approach goes against what the baby's natural instincts are. Typically, when the baby is eating different foods than the rest of the family, they are also fed at a separate time. It is difficult for mom or dad to feed themselves and spoon feed their baby at the same time. In this example, the baby lacks the social interaction that family table time can bring and the opportunity to watch mom, dad, and siblings eat. The infant also loses the chance to examine what they are eating with their hands, eyes, and mouth and explore the family's typical cuisine. Have you ever sat at the zoo and watched chimpanzees interact? I am fascinated by this. There is always one bouncing around while the others sit and stare at their family members, taking it all in. Watch and observe their behavior when you get a chance. Children watch and observe others in this same way. They mostly watch how their parents' conduct themselves to establish what is normal and appropriate behavior. This begins very early. So get the infant around the table the moment they show an interest in food, so you can begin to work on positive associations and interactions with food right away!

As we explore this new concept of introducing food to our baby, we need to be aware that there are definite cues our child gives us to tell us they have had enough. When an infant is nursing, they pull off and sometimes shake their head back and forth and squirm and push away when they are full. With a bottle, they will turn their head away, push their tongue against the nipple to push it out of their mouth, or use their hands to bat the bottle away. They are very smart little cookies.'

Here are some of the cues a baby will give when they do not want to eat. The baby may:

- Turn their head away when they are full or do not want to eat

- Push your hand away

- Try to grab the spoon from your hand

- Spit their food out

- Blow raspberries while eating
- Squirm
- Arch their back to get out of high chair
- Throw their food on the floor and cry
- Shake their head back and forth

Some of the mistakes parents make when feeding their baby include ignoring these cues or second guessing them. They often question whether their child really meant to swat the spoon out of their hands, spit their food out, or turn their head away. So parents continue forking food into their infant's mouth until they gag or no longer can fight. Often I hear parents say "OK, OK, I hear you, you are done." I think, my gosh, it would have been way easier if you had listened the first time. Or they may scold their baby for throwing food on the floor. But how else was their child supposed to tell them they were finished if you weren't catching it the first time?

Parents continue to drum up creative ways to force feed their child (it sounds harsh, but it is true) because they have tried so hard to prepare their food and want their child to eat it and grow from it, or because they have an idea in their mind of how much their baby should eat before they call it quits. So babies are typically spoon fed more in creative ways, leaving the baby crying and parents feeling frustrated and exhausted from facing this feeding frenzy. Many times I have seen parents distract the feeding baby with cheerios and toys on their tray. Parents will also go so far to make helicopter sounds to force one or two more spoonfuls into their child's mouth. Parents often tell me their child eats the best when they are in front of the television. Why? Because the child becomes so distracted by the TV, they are not present with what they are doing and they don't register whether they even want the food or not.

Babies can't talk, so they give you cues. I know it isn't always that easy. It takes a lot of practice for us parents; a completely conscious and present practice to observe and understand the cues your baby is giving. Take this scenario into adulthood, and it's no wonder we can eat a whole bag of potato chips in front of the television without even knowing it, later feeling guilty and bad about it.

Our adult eating behaviors all stem from how food was introduced to us as children, what our dinner table was like, and how our parents approached food with us. So let's make these connections and begin to disconnect from our comfortable place and form a simple technique, which is feeding your baby the food you and the rest of the family are eating and allowing your baby to explore these foods. We need to be present by losing the distractions; cell phones, televisions, and mid-dinner phone calls, to understand and visually observe what our babies' needs are. This is why I strongly recommend the baby-led weaning approach as described above. It takes the frustration away from both the parent and the baby, because now parents can continue their role of simply providing so their baby has the opportunity to explore and eat at their own leisure.

We can and will reestablish better associations and patterning with food and body image so we will forever be out of the jail cell of constant calorie counting, scale hopping, and guilt that is associated with food. So stick with me here as we explore the different age groups and how to make positive changes around your family table.

The Toddler and the Table (One to Three Years Old)

The toddler is an interesting and sometimes frustrating stage of the human cycle. This is one of those stages where control is executed by the little toddler and parents often lose their minds. There is a lot of crying and communication frustrations between parent and their child at this stage. Tantrums develop, and the toddler has a difficult time negotiating, understanding, or seeing your point of view. Well here's a news flash if you haven't already discovered it; your toddler is a lot smarter than you think. And if they were able to get away with it last time, they certainly will bank on getting away with it a second time. And if they can't the second time, they will remember they got away with it once before and continue to display undesirable behavior until the parent breaks this pattern and remains consistent. Their brains are just like little computer banks, absorbing every ounce, taking it all in, watching and learning from their surroundings.

Toddlers are not typically growing much, so their need for food is very little and often comes in spurts. Because of this, this is the time when parents typically will throw in the towel and begin giving in to their toddler. They may go to great lengths to cater and feed their toddler exactly what they want, bringing out the helicopter games, having their child sit on their lap to be fed, and allowing their toddler to get up and down from the table and graze at their choosing. Well this is when everything you learned in the previous chapters goes right out the window. As discussed previously, we know we cannot force our child to eat. So instead of focusing on how much your child is eating, this is the time to instill manners and what to expect from your toddler around the table and to be extremely consistent while doing it. To establish this consistency, you first need to know what you expect from your child and your child needs to be aware of this as well. Then you need to be very consistent with these expectations every single time; offering consequences and reminders for when they are not being met and positive reinforcement and reassurance when they are being met. This will give your toddler an opportunity to understand over and over again what is expected of them.

I was watching my daughter play soccer last night, and the coach on our team praised the girls every time they did something right. Because they are learning the game, they need constant positive reinforcement so they will be motivated enough to make the changes and follow the rules of the game. So our coach chose to focus on all the right stuff, saying such things as, "I love how you are defensive with the ball and how you lean your shoulder into the player to get the ball, great save, awesome kick, wow you run so fast, keep it up girls, you are making amazing saves, high five" He was constantly praising the girls and building them up. This type of parenting or coaching gives the girls positive reinforcement and self confidence when they are doing a lot of things right. And his team showed it by winning games. The girls were motivated and excited, and for the first time, Ryley can't wait to play soccer each week. Meanwhile, the coach on the other team was negative and draining, always pointing out what the girls on his team were doing wrong. I heard "Move over, run faster, stop what you are doing, come on, get out on the field, let's go, why are you doing that, hurry up," and the list goes on. His team was unmotivated, sluggish, continually doing the wrong things and they were losing games.

So when asked what works best, it is positive reinforcement to motivate your child and build self-esteem. Consistency and positive reinforcement when your child is doing something right is what children want and need. When we are consistent in our actions and with our words, life is predictable for our little guys. Think of saying one thing one day and then contradicting what you said the next day. Some days a child gets in trouble for doing something, and other times a parent blows it off like it is no big deal. Or sometimes you count to three and then there are consequences and other times when three is reached there are no consequences. When we are consistent, our children are able to understand what is expected of them and what we need from them. They feel safe, secure, and loved in their environment. They no longer walk on eggshells, waiting for the explosion to happen. We need to carry these consistencies to the table. You will begin to see that consistency around the table enables your child to eat more of what is put in front of them and enjoy it, as well as establish connections with family members around the table. Toddlers wake up every day wanting to have a great day. So it is up to us as parents to help create an environment where they can succeed.

So what does consistency really mean? Consistency is rules and expectations that are the same from one time to another. Consistency makes the child's world predictable and less confusing. It frees their minds of worry about what might happen and teaches them accountability for their actions. Consistency gives a child a sense of security. They learn they can rely on their parents and trust that their needs will be met, helping the bonding process. Children with consistent parents experience less anxiety, and it allows for development of a daily routine with regular rising times, bedtimes, after-school schedules, and meal times to create a more peaceful home life. Consistency helps a child develop a sense of responsibility because they know what their parents expect from them. Children who have consistent rules with predictable consequences are less likely to push the limits and constantly test their parents by misbehaving. They learn quickly that no means no. Invest early in consistent parenting to create considerably fewer temper tantrums, arguing, and bargaining as the child grows.

Through this journey of feeding your children, I need you to be consistent with your child. Children are constantly looking for a place of safety and consistency in how we respond to their actions. And one of the places children and families are struggling constantly is with food and table time. I would like you to develop a foundation of expectations around your dinner table. What is appropriate in your family and what is not? When a foundation is developed at the table, it allows for the basic necessity of food to be eaten in a calm, peaceful, and positive atmosphere. This further facilitates positive growth in your children and the ability for your child to consciously understand what their body needs. When this foundation is not created, children shy away from food, control their negative environment by refusing to eat, starving themselves and later hiding and binge eating in their bedrooms or when nobody is looking. So let's continue to develop this family hub and see how the power of the table can create a new family that connects, grows, and reunites through positive associations with food. Please be firm, be sure your toddler understands what you expect from them at the table, and be consistent. Below are some consistent table etiquette rules that work to establish a positive family table.

Table Time and Etiquette Rules

1. Everyone remains seated at the table until all family members are finished.

2. Please be sure your child is sitting properly, feet off of their chair, and they are turned square toward the table.

3. If your child chooses to forgo eating, please have them come to the table anyway. Serve them a small portion and keep their plate in front of them until everyone is finished. It is important your toddler sees the food that is being served, and you may be surprised that once they discover the table is a safe and positive haven, they may choose to explore.

4. If your child does not like what is being served, simply remind them to politely keep it to themselves and just leave their food on their plate. Think about this, if they were going to your boss's house for dinner and your children decided to announce they didn't like what was

being served, it would be embarrassing for you and hurtful to your boss. So teaching this at home will help to establish appropriate behavior when outside of the home.

5. Keep the conversation away from the food that is being served and keep it focused on positive, light, and fluffy talk. This is a time to talk about how great your day was and share funny stories you may have. This is not a time to discuss marks, or homework, or discipline your child. Keep the conversation light! Make sure everyone is included in the conversation, too. If children do not feel included or do not understand the conversation, they will act out in boredom. So be certain to include everyone at the table.

6. Children can eat as much or as little as they want. If your child would like more, they can have more. For example, if they haven't eaten their peas but would like more rice, they can have more rice. You may decide not to make as much rice next time so you can say, "The rice is all gone, but I have lots of peas, carrots, and corn left if you would like some." Refrain from asking your child to have one more bite of something before they can have more of another food group. This will alleviate ranking foods and keep them all on the same level.

7. Begin to teach appropriate manners and demonstrate how to pass things at the table and how to use cutlery, etc.

8. Get ready for tantrums. This will happen a few times while the rules get into place. For example, if your toddler is used to getting up when they are finished or coming back and forth to the table for a few more bites, the rules now state that they must remain at the table. Give your child a warning that they are no longer able to get up and down from the table because it is distracting for mom, dad, and sister, who are still eating. So if your child is finished and they do not want to sit at the table, then they must go to their room and hang out there instead. The same thing happens when a child acts up at the table. Give them a warning and then they need to be excused and go to their room until the meal is over. This is not meant to be a punishment, so please refrain from raising your voice or getting upset with your child. Rather use a calm voice and explain where they need to go. Sometimes the child will need some help getting to their room as they may flat out refuse. Be patient and assist them. They may also continue to run out of their room and try to get back to the table; continue to put them back in their room. Your mealtime may be destroyed while dealing with this, but trust me, over the next couple of days you will see how calm mealtime will be. When we simply let a child down from the table while the meal is still in play, your child will simply run around, distract other family members, jump

on couches etc. to get your attention and exert their control- "feed me what I want and then I won't be a wild animal around the table." Children would rather hang around the safe hub of the newly established table than in their rooms now that the conversation around the table is light, fluffy and fun.   Over the next couple of days your child will choose to stay at the table and this will facilitate further positive associations with food.

9.   All children must sit on their own chair and not on a parent's lap.

10.   Have each child and parent sit in the same seat each night.

11.   It is very important each family member be served the same meal.

12.   Serve small portions, as large portions can overwhelm a child. One small broccoli tree or one diced carrot, for example.

13.   It takes up to nine exposures of the same food served in the exact same way for a child to try it. And by trying it, I mean attempting to touch it with their fork, smelling it or touching it close to their lips.

14.   Please refrain from talking about their food at the table, such as asking them to take two more bites. Just leave it alone and focus on positive conversations!

15.   A parent's dislike can often spill over onto

their children. When a child sees that daddy doesn't eat broccoli or daddy has announced he doesn't like broccoli, those words and actions speak volumes. Please be sure parents are treated the same as their children. Everyone gets exposed to what is being served on their plate...even daddy (I love how I chose to use dads in this example). Because guess what? It takes daddy up to nine exposures of the same food served in the exact same way before he will eat it, too.

Give your child feedback about expectations as appropriate, such as, "Aiden, please tuck your feet under the table, I would hate for you to fall," or "Please ask to have the butter passed to you instead of reaching over, you may knock something and it makes it a lot easier for mommy to pass it to you," or "I love how nicely you are sitting at the table this evening and your story from school is so funny." Give your child lots of praise and acknowledgement when they meet the expectation and gentle reminders when they need to tweak them. This can be tiresome, but the rewards pay off in all aspects of your parenting life, not just at those times around the table. For example, yesterday, my daughter came home from a friend's house close to bed time, and she immediately wanted help doing her homework. I said, "Sure, I can help you once you get your pajamas on, use the washroom, and brush your teeth." Lately, she has put up a fight with many things, so this is just another one of those scenarios where she was testing the waters and my ability to be consistent. She said she didn't want to put her pajamas on (remember she is seven), and she wanted to wear her clothes to bed. I restated what I needed, saying, "I need your pajamas on, and I need you to use the washroom and brush your teeth before I can help you with your homework."

I love the word "need" because it doesn't allow for any wiggle room. It is firm and assertive and allows me to stay consistent. I explained I was giving her one more chance, otherwise, no homework, and right to bed. NO HOMEWORK—did this mom actually say that? She was testy and again told me she wasn't going to do as I had asked. So I said, "fine, off to bed then." With that, she begged and pleaded that she was sorry. And of course it pulls your heart strings...she told me she needed to get her homework done or her teacher was going to be mad at her. She pulled out all stops to get to me to bargain with her. But remember, consistency is key, and if I want Ryley to listen to me and know I mean what I say, then I need to stand my ground when I say it, regardless of her response or the subject at hand. This may sound crazy to some parents, who might think if your child wants to do homework, even under their parameters, you should grant that. Well no, I mentioned it is important in all aspects of your child's life to be consistent if you want to establish positive relationships with food at the table. If this is one of those times, then so be it. This scenario helps establish rules that your child knows you mean what you say and do as you say. Stand your ground each and every time, regardless of the outcome, situation, or response. At this age, they are learning the norms of what is right and what is wrong and whether mom or dad really mean business. So go out there parents and practice consistency each and everyday!

We have developed a society of the pickiest eaters. It is at this fine age of toddlerhood that likes and dislikes around food are established. Just a slight news flash here, this is all a falsehood. The second we begin to put labels on the foods your child likes and dislikes is the moment your child begins to establish their own parameters around food. And children like to abide by these norms. Remember, they like consistency and they like things to be predictable. So if they tell you they do not like something, they would prefer to never see it again. Well if that was the case they would eat bread and pasta for the rest of their lives. Your child didn't receive the memo that they need to see the same food served in the exact same way nine times before they will even look at it. So of course, right out the gates, it is only normal for your child to turn their nose up at something new.

My rule is never talk about what was eaten or what wasn't eaten. Too much attention around dislikes and likes establishes norms for your child, so we want to refrain from that. One day I made an egg salad sandwich for my daughter's lunch, and I don't know what came over me that day, but I said, "You didn't eat your sandwich today"? I was still in the practicing stage. Bad idea on my part. My daughter said, "Mommy, I don't like egg salad sandwiches. Please never ever pack those in my lunch again...I won't eat it if you do." So I thought, of course I am going to pack it again, is she nuts? Does she know who she is talking to here? I waited a couple of months and tried again. When the lunch bag came back, the sandwich was gone. She had eaten every last morsel of her egg salad sandwich. I couldn't help but open my big fat mouth again. "You ate all of your sandwich this time," I said. "Do you like egg salad sandwiches now?"

Reverting to what she had said before, Madison said, "Mommy, I do not like egg salad sandwiches and I asked you to never ever pack them for me again...I hate them." So case in point, children will keep their word if you allow them to dislike something, and when you keep bringing up what they ate, it gives them negative attention, and they begin to formulate norms around their likes and dislikes. From that day forward, I have never talked about what was or what wasn't eaten from her lunch again. It doesn't matter to me. What matters to me is that my child is being exposed to a variety of different foods to explore and eat at her own leisure. Sometimes her favorite foods are not eaten, so there is no rhyme or reason for what children choose to eat.

Here's another example, which may be very familiar

to you. Your children may not eat carrots at their own house, but when carrots are presented at their friend's house, they eat them all up. Why? Because there is no battle for control at their friend's house, while at home, the battle is on. The child gets a rise out of you and wants to challenge you. Before you fall into this trap...keep your mouth shut. Refrain from talking about what your child eats and doesn't eat, especially because who cares...we know eventually they will try it. My eleven-year-old just ate avocado for the first time a year ago, and only in sushi up to this point. She would never touch it otherwise. But we kept trying. And soon it clicked!

When we label our child as picky (this allows them to be picky). Stop making a million meals to please everyone's palate. No wonder moms are so seriously stressed out. I am telling you right now you can stop catering and follow the etiquette rules of serving the same thing to everyone regardless of past patterns or past tantrums. Remember it is not a child's job to choose what is being served. That is mom and dad's job. To clarify once again, it is going to take your toddler at least nine exposures of the same food, presented in the exact same way, for your child to even attempt to talk about it and then maybe attempt to touch it. Their initial reaction to something new is, "I don't like that." So listen to me here; children establish these likes and dislikes to drive you nuts for one, but also to control you or exert their control over you. And it works! There is nothing your child wants more right now than to be in the driver seat and they will scream, have tantrums, and fall on the ground to get their way. So this is where you need to focus on what we have learned so far. As long as you are offering foods to your child, they have the choice whether they eat that food or not. More often than not, your child will eat one day, and avoid that food they loved the next day. So don't overthink it; there is no pattern here whatsoever, and this is why these concrete rules offer a simple, consistent solution to guide you to creating a positive family table.

School Age Children and the Table

We teach ourselves to be mindful by teaching ourselves to be awake and aware of what we are doing. We also want to teach this to our children. Let them understand when they want to eat, try something new, or leave their food for another time. Allow them to be mindful of how they feel, when they need fuel, and when they do not. My five-year-old spent a whole year not eating her dinner, and it was funny because I never even noticed until I actually reflected on it. It doesn't even appear on my radar screen. I lose zero sleep if she decides she doesn't want to eat. Now, at seven, she still isn't a huge dinner eater. By the end of the day, she is tired and has gotten all of her food in from breakfast, snacks, and lunch. She loves the dinner table though, because we have built a connection and fun time with great conversation.

I have a funny story. On occasion, I will serve turkey chili. Each time I served turkey chili to my five-year-old, she would say she didn't like it, but she knew the drill that she needed to come to the table. She would be sure to warn me before she sat down at the table that she wasn't going to eat it. So in my head, I thought here we go again, bite my tongue, be consistent, and say, "That's fine, you don't have to eat it." I teach this stuff; I can do this again.

Why did I do this?

1. Because now, at seven years old, my daughter eats bowls of turkey chili without a fuss. When a child is exposed to the same dish many times, and a parent doesn't budge to give them what they want instead; they will eventually try it.

2. There is no such thing as not liking something.

3. To be consistent and follow the rule; parents provide and children choose whether they will eat it or not and how much.

4. Because she sat at the table and joined in on our conversation that bonds our family together. It is the one time we don't talk about

what foods we like and what foods we don't like, but rather is a time to connect about our day and deepen our relationships with each other. It's a time to feel safe around the hub of the table.

5.   She was able to see other family members enjoying the turkey chili several times and the fact that none of us died from it was encouraging to her. This was helpful in leading her down the road to trying it too.

6.   I didn't force my daughter to eat it, or bribe or reward her for taking a bite, allowing her to establish positive relationships with food. There were no strings attached.

I would serve the smallest of bowls to my daughter. When children are trying something for the first time or you are serving them something they do not typically eat, it is important to serve small portions. One cube of carrot, one stem of broccoli, or one tablespoon of turkey chili. I even put it in a smaller bowl or on a smaller plate. When serving sizes are large, they are very overwhelming, and your child will get discouraged quickly. For example, when my daughter did eat her tablespoon of chili, she was so happy because she could see that it was all gone in her bowl, despite the serving size. The next time, I will serve one tablespoon more.

The Teenager ... the Importance of Table Time

This is the age when your child has an opinion and can begin to make their own choices...it is difficult to nail down a teenager, between school, jobs, friends, and activities, and you may find their eating patterns difficult to track. Often they skip breakfast, eat on the fly, and pack in food at friends' houses or fast-food joints when their body calls out in hunger. So when dinner is being served, they may be full, but after dinner they may be up making food in the kitchen again. This is their way of gaining their own independence and their bodies are also growing in a lot of strange and new ways, so it is all good, although it can be frustrating for the parent who has prepared a dinner meal. If we go back to what we have learned in previous chapters, the table is for connecting, it is a place that brings the family together for positive conversation, so it is important that regardless of hunger or fullness, you encourage your teenager to come to the table. Just like we did with the toddler and school age child, we want to continue with the teenager, too. They do not have to eat, but you would like to connect with them. So simply have them join you at the table. Quite frankly for most this is the only time you will converse with your teenager and continue to build a connection.

At this stage, the parent still gets to control what is being served. I always say to my children, "Until you have a paycheck and are buying groceries, I get to choose what food I spend my money on." If that sounds too harsh to say (although it is true), then just believe it. At this age, your child can start to contribute to meal time. Make a list of meals you enjoy with your teenager, and have them cook a meal or two for the family. This is an amazing way to get your teenager into the kitchen, and if they are cooking and spending their time on a meal, they will be sure to eat it too. If you are working late or want a night off from cooking, allow your teenager to whip up their favorite meal for the family.

Try to keep meal times the same each night, so your teenager knows what to expect and can hold off and wait. Give them some responsibility of saving their money so they are not spending it all on fast food. This will allow them to appreciate a home-cooked meal. As dinner becomes more consistent in your household, you will begin to notice that your teenager comes to the table hungry and participates in your fluffy and fun conversation.

The Spouse and the Table ... Just Like Children

Sometimes our spouses can be like children. They can be as tough, if not tougher than the rest of the family to feed. The older they get, the harder it is to change old habits. We are built on familiar norms that we adapted to growing up, and we continue to stick to those routines and rituals around the table. If television was watched while eating as a child, we often continue to follow this pattern into adulthood. So to make this system work, it is important that both mom and dad adhere to the new family rules. One time, I blew it and made the mistake of getting up to wash dishes before everyone was done. From that day forward, I knew I needed to set a good example for my children. Refrain from jumping up and answering the phone, running off to a meeting, or checking e-mails while eating. Engage in conversation with your children that is stimulating and something they can understand. The family table is a really fun place!

11 WHAT TO FEED YOUR FAMILY

Beverages, Anyone?

Did somebody say water? Yes, I did. H2O it is. Water offers so many benefits without providing a caloric load leading to fullness. So if you want your child to feel hunger, serve them water only. You may hear some complaints from the peanut gallery when you start this routine, but if you follow the rules, everything will begin to fall into place. You will see. In our family, we use a tall glass bottle that gets filled with water straight from the tap every day for lunch and dinner meals. I leave cups at the table, so the children can fill their cup up as they choose, and, voila, everyone is pouring and enjoying!

What About Juice and Milk?

As a parent, you may wonder about milk. Milk is full of calories, but also contains nutrients that are beneficial to your child's growth and development. So serve organic milk at breakfast if you desire, or in between meal times, and stick to water for your lunch and dinner meal.

Juice is just a filler. Although it may indicate it contains wonderful nutrients on the bottle, juice is made from the bruised, battered, and sometimes moldy and rotten fruits at the orchard. The fruit is boiled at high temperatures to kill bacteria, and is then bottled. Some juices contain many preservatives to sustain shelf life and prevent growth of mold and bacteria. At the end of the day, juice contains very little nutrients and has high sugar content. Even though sugar isn't listed as an ingredient on the label, fruit naturally contains sugars that act in the same way as white sugar in the body. So to avoid additional sugars in your child's diet, it's easy, just take the juice out.

Snacks After Dinner?

Did somebody say fruit? Yes, I did. The only item that is served after dinner is fruit. That's it. So after dinner is cleaned up and my children have bathed and have their jammies on, they may have fruit. In our home, I purchase the fruit that is on sale at the local grocery store that week. So if watermelon is on sale, watermelon is an option. At that time, my children may have as much watermelon as they would like. There are no limits to the portion of fruit. Some parents indicate that their children do not like fruit, but again, I would still offer this as the only option, or you can package up their leftover dinner and allow them a second chance at it. Once you stick to this routine, you will begin to see that one, they actually do like fruit, and two, they eat their dinner.

What About Dessert?

Get rid of dessert altogether while you establish your family table. For one, children do not need dessert every night. Two, this takes the pressure off of bribing or rewarding for finished food, so there is nothing to dangle in front of your child's face with comments such as, "Well, I have a great dessert if you eat your meal," or "Look, David ate all of his dinner so he is going to get dessert, but you won't." The third reason to take dessert away is it gets your child eating at their own free will, knowing there is nothing else coming. It will take you a few months to start to see definite results. It takes persistence and consistency. I suggest keeping dessert outside of the home, such as a special ice cream cone midday, or a walk to the local convenience store for a freezie or a dessert when you go out for dinner. This way nobody in the family is tempted by cookies and ice cream. When dessert is being served in the home, buy just enough and serve it very occasionally, so dessert isn't expected.

On the off chance that dessert is being served, everyone in your household can enjoy dessert regardless of how they ate their dinner. Taking dessert away for a while is the best scenario while establishing the family table.

What Do I Serve My Child Between Meals?

Here is a list of great snacks that can be served to any age child between meals. Please refrain from serving snacks too close to meal times. I suggest a cut off of two hours before meals. Snacks should be served between breakfast and lunch and between lunch and dinner, and fruit is to be served after dinner, as discussed earlier. Clean any snacks that are not on this list out of your home. Simply take a garbage bag and pitch them, or donate unused snacks to the local food bank. This is a very important step in feeding your children properly.

Here is a list of snacks I recommend having in your household:

SNACKS

- Full fat yogurt (organic preferred, any flavor)
- Roasted chickpeas with gentle seasoning to taste
- Hummus with rice crackers, kasha crackers, bread sticks, or veggies, or put into a wrap with red peppers
- 2%–4% cottage cheese
- White brick cheese, cubed
- Soft cheese or goat's cheese spread on crackers or celery
- Mashed avocado mixed with hummus for dipping or spread on a wrap or pita
- Unsweetened applesauce
- Dry cereal (head to the health food section of your local grocery store and pick one out)
- Kale chips
- Roasted seaweed
- Boiled egg
- Nut-free trail mix (pumpkin seeds, sunflower seeds, carob chips, raisins)
- Rice cakes, corn thins, or rice crackers with natural peanut butter or almond butter
- Natural unsalted tortilla chips with salsa

- Homemade pita chips
- Edamame beans

Will My Child Starve?

It is normal for parents to initially worry that their children will starve if they are not fed what they like. This is why we ended up here in the first place. It comes from a loving place, where parents want to provide whatever they can so their children will grow. Your child will not starve. They will never starve; I can promise you. Your child will starve, however, if you continue to pattern negative experiences around the table.

When you initiate the new rules, your child may not eat a lot the first day, but over the next couple of days, you will notice their appetite increase and their liking for food increases, too. When you take all of the between meal and after-dinner junk out, you will see how things change. In previous chapters, I discussed how smart our bodies are and how they know exactly how much food we need. So continue to trust this philosophy, and free yourself from the controlling feelings that your child won't grow, will starve, or will grow too much!

What About Breakfast and Lunch?

I want you to focus on the table etiquette rules for dinner because that is the one meal where most families are able to sit down together as a unit. Although, if you find another meal easier for you, then that works just as well. In some families where the father works late hours or in a single parent home, one parent having dinner with their children is just as effective as both. The more opportunity you have to sit together as a family, the more chances you will have to develop a positive family table.

In our home, I am able to eat lunch with our children during the summer months, and on weekends, I plan all three meals with the family. For breakfast during the school year, I allow my children to choose what they want and they can eat at the breakfast counter while I prepare their school lunches. Because all of my kids get ready for school at different rates, with the end result of leaving the house at the same time, I allow them to manage their time in the morning and get down from the table when they are finished.

Helping Out in the Kitchen

Begin getting your children into the kitchen and helping out. I have my daughters peel carrots, stir up pancake mix, make mac and cheese, flip pancakes, put together hamburgers, and this year, they made their teachers banana bread for Christmas by following a recipe. Giving them this opportunity creates a bonding experience and teaches them how much fun, and how much work, cooking can be, too. This takes a lot of patience on the parents' part, but over time, you will find that they offer you a lot of help.

Get them to set the table, clear the table, or fold the napkins. Anything that brings the family together to prepare the meal. Last summer, we got a pizza oven for our backyard, and it has been fantastic for bringing our family together. We play outside while the oven heats up and watch the fire after our pizzas have been cooked. We have the chance to make the pizzas to our liking and watch them cook. There is something about cooking and eating together that brings us closer.

12 LEARN FROM MISTAKES

Let go of your control over your children, and let them learn from their mistakes. If a child cannot make a mistake, they will never learn from that experience. Take a baby who is learning to walk, they fall and get up again a million times a day. Each time, they learn from their mistakes, and eventually take their first step on their own using what they've learned. Parents often smother, protect, and enable their children by controlling the outcome of their children's experiences, growth, and choices. Enabling occurs when we help to rescue our children from their own problems instead of letting them deal with the consequences. It can also include taking over their tasks, bailing them out when they get into trouble, or allowing them to get away with things instead of making them accountable for their actions.

We choose to clean up our children's messes, always protecting them from failure, because we do not trust that our children can make age appropriate decisions and experience failure and disappointment. Failure and disappointment are the key elements of allowing your children to learn, problem solve, and become self-sufficient individuals.

Here are some examples. Giving your child more money when they spend all their allowance so they can have money to go out with their friends. Another example is doing homework for your child to ensure they get good grades. A third example is giving in to your child's every desire and whim because you can't stand seeing them upset. And a fourth example is feeding your children exactly the foods they want so they do not starve (I offer this word lightly), get upset, or cause a scene at the table.

This rut parents have gotten themselves into is meant to control the outcome of their child's efforts. But what happens when the parent is no longer around at the next party where there are drugs and alcohol? Or the first time they could be confronted to have intercourse? What happens then? The child has always been protected and sheltered from ever having a bad experience. And if they make a bad choice their parents will further bail them out so they suffer few consequences. I know we have jumped from food choices to sex, but every experience sets your child up for success or failure. When they fail is when they succeed. The most successful people make mistakes. In children who are enabled, there are more cases of substance abuse and psychological problems down the road. These children are not as driven and not as successful as those who have had to work through their problems and suffered the consequences of their actions.

The cold weather hit our town of Oakville ON and my seven year old Ryley...soon to be eight (cry face) left for school; she leaves the house before her older sister and walks on her own to school now (double cry face). She wants to be on time! As she was leaving I noticed she didn't have her hat or mitts on. I asked her if she needed her hats and mitts today and she said, "no I'm fine." I prompted again, "are you sure?" and she replied "yes I am sure, " and off she went.

Meanwhile later that morning I stepped outside to discover how cold it had become. My first response to myself was "Oh no, Ryley went to school without her mitts and hat, she is going to freeze to death". Then I stopped and thought about how long her breaks outside were and what I would do if I had forgot my hat and mitts. I thought how she would likely put her hood up, run around to stay warm and tuck her hands into her jacket.

Now I work from home, so I can easily drop mitts and hats by the school. But I stopped myself, "Wait a minute here. She isn't going to freeze to death. Yes, she will feel pain from the cold but how is she going to learn what she needs to bring to school in the morning if she doesn't feel the cold?" Ah ... the guilt set in, from thoughts of what are the other parents going to think and what about the teachers if they see her with no hat and mitts, what kind of a mom are they going to think I am. And then the guilt left and I just let it go.

I need and want to raise children that make mistakes and learn from them. I know we only grow when we make mistakes. If I constantly told Ryley she needed her hat and mitts or forced her to put them on, I would be doing this every single morning until April. So when Ryley came running through the door after school she shouted "I am FREEZING" I said, "I know it is so cold out there!" I then asked her, what she could do differently tomorrow to keep herself warm. She told me what she would do and today she was all dressed and ready for school with her snow pants on, winter boots, hat, gloves and a scarf. No prompting from me at all ;)

Enabling and controlling as parents feels like the right direction to help a child, but in fact it is actually enabling them rather than empowering them to be successful and responsible children, teens, and adults. I take my husband as an example. He had to get a job in ninth grade to pay for his wants, and each summer, he worked mowing lawns and running a painting company. In eighth grade his family could not afford to send him on his school trip. So when high school came and a trip to Quebec City presented itself, he worked extra hard to pay for it and joined his classmates. In his last two weeks of university, he ran out of money entirely, but instead of asking for money from his parents, he began to sell his belongings—baseball cards, CDs, etc., to get by. Now he has a very successful career. He learned what it takes to take care of himself. He went from broke (running out of money, which for some is seen as failure) to working hard to make money. Did you know Donald Trump has filed for bankruptcy four times in his life? And Walt Disney lived in his office and ate beans from a can to get his business up and running; also filed bankruptcy. We have got to learn from our mistakes in order to move ourselves forward.

Enabling our children by feeding them what they want so they won't starve doesn't allow them to experience what their body really needs. Enabling our children by bribing them with reward never lets them experience consequences. And enabling our children by force feeding never lets them make choices. Trust that your child knows what they need and how much they need at every step along the way. The positive environment will continue to develop and the root of your family table will flourish.

13 YOUR FAMILY DINNER PLAN

Week One:

Choose six dinner meals you currently make for your Family.

Step One

To get these strategies on the road, we need to start with dinner and take small steps to get different foods on the table. First, I would like you to write down six meals your family currently enjoys. If you do not enjoy meals as a family, for example children eat chicken fingers and fries and parents eat steak, vegetables, and salad, you will need to compromise with a meal you can all enjoy together. So you may decide that one night it is chicken fingers and fries and the next night it is steak, vegetables, and rice or corn on the cob. Please list your meals here:

1.

2.

3.

4.

5.

6.

Step Two

Take a journal and fit the above six meals into the evenings that work with your schedule. Base it around who is home and who can cook and whether you have extra activities in the evenings. In my plan, I keep the cooking simple on the evenings we have soccer and I save the prep of more extravagant meals for the evenings we are at home. Spread your planning over two weeks if you find you need more days.

Example Journal	*Mon*	*Tue*	*Wed*	*Thu*	*Fri*	*Sat*	*Sun*
Breakfast							
• Snack 1							
• Snack 2							
Lunch							
• Today's activities							
• Who's home for dinner?							
Dinner							
• What can I add to dinner this week?							
Result							

You can also download a pdf version of a journal at www.highwaytohealth.ca

Week Two:

I would like you to take the meals you cooked last week and add a twist to each of the meals. This is a very small twist. For example, chicken fingers and fries could be changed to homemade breaded chicken and fries or chicken fingers and potatoes, vegetable, or white rice. You may switch white rice to brown rice, or mix a touch of brown rice into your white rice. Or instead of white potatoes, add in a few pieces of sweet potato, too. Or add an additional vegetable to your meal. If you were making frozen hamburger patties, make your patties from scratch this week. Or with pasta sauce, add a splash of spinach or add a touch of ground beef to tomato sauce. Make small changes this week and include these new changes into a new journal, basing your meals around the activities you have planned for the week.

Week Three:

Continue this pattern of tweaking your meals to become healthier options for your family. In addition, this week, I would like you to add a meal into the rotation that you LOVE. Not what others like, but one that you enjoy, and begin to add this meal into your routine. If you are unsure of a meal, use a recipe book or google a recipe online to use. Some find it is a success based on the structure that we have created, and others find this new meal addition is a bust, but a much better bust than how meal time looked before. Continue to rotate this meal into the mix every one to two weeks so your children can begin to get some exposure to this meal.

It is around this time you may be getting sick of your meals. If grilled cheese, chicken fingers, and eggs on toast were family favorites, you could be getting tired of these meals; but keep tweaking, and each week add in a new flare to your menu. With the new fare, you can begin to wean out the meals that are not so good. Instead, you could serve eggs and toast for breakfast and eat as a family. This slow transition helps your child see familiar foods in addition to the introduction of new foods.

Week Four:

Cook less by rolling over your meals. This week, when you cook your meals, double or quadruple the recipe. For example, if spaghetti sauce was something your family enjoyed, then I would like you to make it into four meals, and use labeled plastic freezer bags to freeze into additional meals. Or if hamburgers are a staple, make a bunch of them to have on hand in the freezer. Now you can use your staple meals for busy nights because you can just pull them out of the freezer. We freeze everything from leftover steak to rollover into a stir fry, to cooked fish to rollover into fish tacos. My rollover nights are easy dinner nights for me. Now plan in your journal what your meals will look like. Bulk up on meals when you have time to cook, and begin stockpiling your freezer. You can follow my rollover meal ideas on Facebook. Go to www.highwaytohealth.ca to connect.

14 NUTRIENTS FOR OUR KIDS

What Nutrients Do Children Need More Of?

PROTEIN

- Meat protein (Chicken, beef, pork, turkey, lamb, two eggs, five ounces of lamb)
- Fish/seafood (Tuna, salmon, fresh or frozen fillets, shrimp)
- Vegetable protein (Five ounces of tofu, veggie burgers, edamame beans)
- Dairy-based protein (Cottage cheese, full fat yogurt, white brick cheese, goat cheese)
- Beans and grains (Hummus, beans, lentils, quinoa)
- Nuts and seeds (Unroasted nuts and seeds, nut butters, tahini)

ESSENTIAL FATTY ACIDS

Walnuts, ground flaxseed, pecans, pine nuts, wheat germ, hemp, pumpkin seeds, spinach, brussels sprouts, soy products, avocados, certain vegetable oils such as canola, grape seed, and olive oil.

IRON

Eggs, fish, leafy green vegetables, whole grains, enriched breads and cereals, almonds, avocados, beets, blackstrap molasses, kidney and lima beans, lentils, peaches, pears, dried fruit, rice, sesame seeds, soybeans, red meat, poultry.

CALCIUM

Milk, cheese, yogurt, salmon, sardines, seafood, dark green leafy vegetables, almonds, asparagus, broccoli, cabbage, collards, oats, tofu, yogurt, goat cheese, tahini, hummus.

What Nutrients Do Children Need Less of?

It is important to avoid the substances below, as they block the consumption of nutritiously rich food.

MONOSODIUM GLUTAMATE (MSG)

Found in soups, mixes, crackers, chips, prepared foods, and dips.

ASPARTAME

Found in sweetened items, Jell-O, yogurts, and fat free/sugar free items.

SUGAR

Primarily found in juices, baked goods, sweets, and sauces.

CHEMICALS

If you cannot pronounce/understand what is on the ingredient list of a label, then your body cannot understand it either, and therefore it should not be consumed.

FOOD COLORING

Found in most juices, freezies, yogurts, and kids' snack

items.

HYDROGENATED VEGETABLE OILS

Contain trans-fatty acids that are detrimental to our health. Found in chips, crackers, doughnuts, french fries, pies, meat pies, fried fish, and chicken fingers. Check out the label and if it is contained in the product it will be indicated on the ingredient list.

15 THE FAMILY HUB

I want you to give yourself a big pat on the back. First, for acknowledging how important the family connection is for you and your children, and second, for taking the time out of your busy life to learn more, be better, and develop a stronger connection to your children. You have begun the process of breaking the emotional eating cycle that once consumed your family's life or the life of someone you know. As you step out and begin to implement these techniques in your family, remember you will do the cha-cha dance. Some days you will take a few steps forward, and other days a few steps back. I ask that you look at the bigger picture, keep a positive outlook, and focus on where you have come from. Sometimes, small changes can be so difficult to see and are forgotten. When you look at what your child was eating a year ago and the connection your family hub had or didn't have a year ago, you will see great strides toward happy, healthier family connections and more solidarity toward positive relationships with food, body image, and how your children use food for growth and nourishment. Continue to be consistent and make these small changes. Your determination and understanding that every child grows at their own pace, in their own time, and in different ways will push you further toward letting go and believing you are doing the right thing. When each family begins to make these positive connections with food, we step further away from measuring our day based on the number on the scale or how we look on the outside, and move closer to turning inward and measuring our day based on how we feel on the inside. The more you continue to have positive connections around the dinner table, the closer you will get to building positive relationships with food for you and your children.

Furthermore, as these positive connections toward food grow around your family table, you will also experience deeper connections and more meaningful relationships with your children and your spouse that are based on trust, love, and respect. A family who laughs together, shares together, and eats together is a family who stays together. Let's get these little guys loving themselves for all of the wonderful things that are going on inside them, and their outer beauty will shine like a bright star. Bodies are truly amazing vehicles, and if we could actually see all of the great things our bodies do each and every day, the emotions they take on, and the thoughts they carry to produce creative uniqueness and beauty in each of us, we would forever look on the inside before we worried about how we or others looked on the outside. Let's keep the focus on healthy, strong, and nourished bodies.

Just the other day, my seven-year-old was typing up a note on the computer. This is exactly what she wrote, and how it looked:

That is why I love my family!!!!!!!

i love my family because?

They are so so so so so so nice to me and my family.

They are so so so so awesome too!!

i love madi!

i love daddy!

i love mommy! and chris!

i love myself!

i love steven and andy too!!!!!

This is not my whole family is

g.g nanny and poppa there is a lot of people in my family. i can't even remEMber who's in my family or not That is why I love my family!!!!!!!

What got me was that she said she loved herself. It was essential to be on the list of people she loved. I know from my practice that not many adults can say they love themselves, so to see my daughter say she does was all I needed to assure me we are doing the right thing as parents. Teaching your children to love themselves! Is that not what we want for each of our children? To love everything about themselves and to be comfortable in their own bodies. To not worry about what people think or say, and to know that we have the best darn body. When we love ourselves, our children can learn how to love themselves through our example. To activate this process for yourself, I would like you to write down three things you like about yourself each and every day. It could be anything from your eyes to how you responded to your friend or that you helped a friend; whatever it may be. But it needs to be three things about only you. See how this gratitude begins to shape how you feel about yourself.

Now go out in this world and build your family table. Build it each and every day. Take pride in the fact that with each meal, you are developing stronger bonds and connections with your children toward a positive body image, self love, and a better relationship with food. No longer is food controlling us. We are in control of what our body needs and wants. Just listen and your body will tell you so.

I would like to personally thank you for taking action to push society forward toward focusing on who we are on the inside. To develop children that shine so bright with their own inner light and to teach them that life is limitless. We are as smart as everyone else who makes up this world we live in. So go out there and continue to create an environment for your family where the table is an especially safe haven where nourishment happens and good things come true!

THE END

FOOTNOTES

webmd.com by Kathleen Doherty, Clutter Control, Is Too Much Stuff Draining You?

webmd.com by Kathleen Doherty, Clutter Control, Is Too Much Stuff Draining You?

ABOUT THE AUTHOR

Roslyn Fisher is a Registered Nutritional Consulting Practitioner (RNCP) and a member of the IONC. She has been practicing nutrition since 2005 through the business she founded Highway to Health or "H2H". Through H2H, Roslyn has helped thousands of individual clients and corporate clients improve their own personal and their families' health and wellness. Today, Roslyn continues to run weight loss and family nutrition programs through H2H. Roslyn is also a mother of two, a step-mom to another two, a life coach and an accomplished public speaker, making many appearances each year.

Visit H2H online at www.highwaytohealth.ca